THE BEST PLACE

MEDICAL ANTHROPOLOGY: HEALTH, INEQUALITY, AND SOCIAL JUSTICE

Series editor: Lenore Manderson

Books in the Medical Anthropology series are concerned with social patterns of and social responses to ill health, disease, and suffering, and how social exclusion and social justice shape health and healing outcomes. The series is designed to reflect the diversity of contemporary medical anthropological research and writing and will offer scholars a forum to publish work that showcases the theoretical sophistication, methodological soundness, and ethnographic richness of the field.

Books in the series may include studies on the organization and movement of peoples, technologies, and treatments, how inequalities pattern access to these, and how individuals, communities, and states respond to various assaults on well-being, including from illness, disaster, and violence.

For a list of all the titles in the series, please see the last page of the book.

THE BEST PLACE

Addiction, Intervention, and Living and Dying Young in Vancouver

DANYA FAST

RUTGERS UNIVERSITY PRESS
New Brunswick, Camden, and Newark, New Jersey
London and Oxford

Rutgers University Press is a department of Rutgers, The State University of New Jersey, one of the leading public research universities in the nation. By publishing worldwide, it furthers the University's mission of dedication to excellence in teaching, scholarship, research, and clinical care.

Library of Congress Cataloging-in-Publication Data

Names: Fast, Danya, author.
Title: The best place : addiction, intervention, and living and dying young in Vancouver / Danya Fast.
Description: New Brunswick, New Jersey : Rutgers University Press, [2024] | Series: Medical anthropology | Includes bibliographical references and index.
Identifiers: LCCN 2023009496 | ISBN 9781978834880 (paperback ; alk. paper) | ISBN 9781978834897 (hardback ; alk. paper) | ISBN 9781978834903 (epub) | ISBN 9781978834927 (pdf)
Subjects: LCSH: Drug addicts—British Columbia—Vancouver—Case studies. | Drug addiction—Treatment—British Columbia—Vancouver—Case studies. | Youth—Drug use—British Columbia—Vancouver—Case studies. | Youth—British Columbia—Vancouver—Social conditions—Case studies.
Classification: LCC HV5840.C32 V3365 2024 | DDC 362.29/30971128—dc23/eng/20230627
LC record available at https://lccn.loc.gov/2023009496

A British Cataloging-in-Publication record for this book is available from the British Library.

References to internet websites (URLs) were accurate at the time of writing. Neither the author nor Rutgers University Press is responsible for URLs that may have expired or changed since the manuscript was prepared.

♾ The paper used in this publication meets the requirements of the American National Standard for Information Sciences—Permanence of Paper for Printed Library Materials, ANSI Z39.48-1992.

rutgersuniversitypress.org

For Rayna
     Lee
     Jordan
     Laura
     Tom
     Terry
     Dom
     Cody
     Carly
     and Patty

CONTENTS

FOREWORD

LENORE MANDERSON

The Medical Anthropology: Health, Inequality, and Social Justice series is concerned with the diversity of contemporary medical anthropological research and writing. The beauty of ethnography is its capacity, through storytelling, to make sense of suffering as a social experience and to set it in context. Central to our focus in this series, therefore, is the way in which social structures, political and economic systems, and ideologies shape the likelihood and impact of infections, injuries, bodily ruptures and disease, chronic conditions and disability, treatment and care, and social repair and death.

Health and illness are social facts: the circumstances of the maintenance and loss of health are always and everywhere shaped by structural, local, and global relations. Social formations and relations, culture, economy, and political organization as much as ecology shape experiences of illness, disability, and disadvantage. The authors of the monographs in this series are concerned centrally with health and illness, healing practices, and access to care, but in the different volumes the authors highlight the importance of such differences in context as expressed and experienced at individual, household, and wider levels. Health risks and outcomes of social structure and household economy (for example, health systems factors), as well as national and global politics and economics, all shape people's lives. In their accounts of health, inequality, and social justice, the authors move across social circumstances, health conditions, geography, and their intersections and interactions to demonstrate how individuals, communities, and states manage assaults on people's health and well-being.

As medical anthropologists have long illustrated, the relationships between social context and health status are complex. In addressing these questions, the authors in this series showcase the theoretical sophistication, methodological rigor, and empirical richness of the field, while expanding a map of illness, social interaction, and institutional life to illustrate the effects of material conditions and social meanings in troubling and surprising ways. The books reflect medical anthropology as a constantly changing field of scholarship, drawing on research in such diverse contexts as residential and virtual communities, clinics, laboratories, and emergency care and public health settings; with service providers, individual healers, and households; and with social bodies, human bodies, biologies, and biographies. While medical anthropology once concentrated on systems of healing, particular diseases, and embodied experiences, today the field has expanded to include environmental disasters, war, science, technology, faith, gender-based violence, and forced migration. Curiosity about the body and its vicissitudes remains a pivot of our work, but our concerns are with the location of bodies in social life and with how social structures, temporal imperatives, and shifting exigencies shape life courses. This dynamic field reflects the ethics of the discipline to address these pressing issues of our time.

As the subtitle of the series indicates, the books center on social exclusion and inclusion, social justice and repair. The volumes in this series illustrate multiple ways in which globalization and national and local inequalities shape health experiences and outcomes across space; economic, political, and social inequalities influence the likelihood of poor health and its outcomes in different settings. At the same time, social and economic relations enable the institutionalization of poverty; they produce the unequal conditions of everyday life and work, and hence, also, of who gets sick and who is most likely to survive. The books challenge readers to reflect on suffering, deficit, and despair within families and communities, while they also encourage readers to remain alert to resistance and restitution—to consider how people respond to injustices and evade the fissures that might seem to predetermine their lives.

Each decade has its own declared "epidemic" of drug (mis)use and associated deaths, depending on what is available, what is licit, and what is not: phenacetin, cannabis, heroin, cocaine, benzodiazepines, methamphetamine, oxycodone, fentanyl. Household and other everyday products are repurposed as drugs to sharpen, muffle, or distort perception: petrol, glue, paint thinner. In response, communities of users, public health workers, medical professionals, and government employees continually sway between criminalization and harm reduction as they attempt to manage the war on drugs and prevent associated harms and deaths. In cities where people congregate to buy, sell, and use drugs and to find others willing to share the pleasures and risks and reciprocate with care, local governments explore a variety of interventions while struggling to identify long-term policies to avoid new waves of harms and casualties. This is the case worldwide; the difference is between states that are willing to respond with compassion and those that vigorously pursue policies of drug prohibition, policing, and incarceration.

Vancouver, located on the Pacific Ocean, is one of Canada's warmest cities, and so while the weather is inclement from other geographic perspectives, it provides refuge for large numbers of people without homes or adequate incomes. Many of these are young people who use drugs, attracted to Vancouver by the city's self-promotion as one of the world's most desirable locales, if also the site of some of the starkest poverty in Canada. Here, as Danya Fast describes in *The Best Place: Addiction, Intervention, and Living and Dying Young in Vancouver*, they struggle to make a home, to build and sustain friendships and romances, and to hold on to imagined futures that are not overdetermined by drugs, violence, and loss.

As we read in this superb and original ethnography, dangerous drug use among young people in Vancouver is an effect not cause of homelessness, poverty, and alienation. Central to how they speak of the challenges of extracting themselves from drugs, they focus on the most proximate driver, that of boredom. Boredom is endemic for young people with incomplete educations, without credentials or skills that might provide them with meaningful jobs, with poor health, and with deep histories of violence associated with unsettled families, torn communities, and racist state policies. As *The Best Place* illustrates, many of those unhomed in the city are Indigenous. Their immediate histories are often accounts of endless foster home placements and other forms of dislocation tied to First Nations, Inuit, and Métis dispossession, displacement, and abandonment.

The Best Place is concerned, centrally, with the everyday rhythms of young people's lives over a dozen years. The first accounts of Fast's protagonists and friends are from 2008; some are still alive in 2020. Other are not; they have overdosed as a result of a drug supply made highly toxic by illicitly-manufactured fentanyl and related analogues. Between first meeting and their untimely deaths, how they live tells us much about what it means to be assigned to the social, spatial, and economic margins of the city, even when living in its geographic and economic center, in decrepit housing tucked behind tourist hotels and elegant restaurants. Young people live without occupations, dependent on state welfare support and constrained by those who determine their rights to such basic support as shelter. How their lives are protected, through allocation to shelter and barely sufficient resources, is deeply problematic. Many cling to ideas of a markedly better, conventional future, as they struggle with the residues of settler colonialism, entrenched poverty, and poor health. A few break away, leaving Vancouver altogether or simply living away from state regimentation—in tents, under bridges, or, temporarily, in family homes.

Fast writes powerfully and evocatively of everyday life and death, substance use, and care. In doing so, she breaks with convention and opts for many short chapters, some just a paragraph long, depicting a single conversation or a chance encounter or event that, storied, draws us deep into the lives of young people. We follow them in *The Best Place* as they ricochet between emergency cold-weather shelters, run-down single room occupancy hotels, rigidly governed supportive housing facilities, drug treatment settings, and beyond. Text is juxtaposed with image, with photographs taken by some of those with whom she worked. Through this break with form and structure, we follow the eddies of despair and dependence of young people's lives and the compassion and creativity that are offered as ways of caring. In this extraordinary book, we build friendships with Fast's young friends, and their deaths are as shocking for us as readers as for her. Such shock opens doors for us all to rethink how best to provide care and save lives, and how to repair the ruptures to social life and well-being that anticipate addiction and the heightened risk of death.

ACKNOWLEDGMENTS

This book is for all of the young people who have given me their time and stories over the past fifteen years. Thank you for bearing with me and explaining and re-explaining, cracking jokes and disagreeing fiercely, and always keeping me safe. You taught me so many important lessons, and I hope that I have done justice to some of them here. I am also grateful to the dedicated group of providers and managers who supported this project in innumerable ways. Any errors are mine alone.

To my other teachers, in particular Thomas Kerr, Jeannie Shoveller, and Dara Culhane, thank you for giving me the words, ideas, and encouragement I needed as this project unfolded. Andrea López, Kelly Knight, Jeff Shonberg, Tyler McCreary, Eileen Moyer, Rob Lorway, Dave Cunningham, and Kali-olt Sedgemore have also been crucial interlocutors over the years. Thank you to Sam Fenn, Garth Mullins, and the Crackdown podcast team; I began collaborating with you just in time to learn several invaluable lessons about how to tell these kinds of stories. My editors Lenore Manderson and Kimberly Guinta were endlessly patient and enthusiastic over the many years that this book was in the making. Thank you for helping me to see it through. I also want to thank the two anonymous reviewers whose insights greatly improved the book.

I am part of a wonderful group of scholars at the British Columbia Centre on Substance Use (BCCSU) and Division of Social Medicine at the University of British Columbia (UBC). Thank you to Evan Wood, Cheyenne Johnson, Will Small, Lindsey Richardson, MJ Milloy, Kanna Hayashi, Mint Ti, Eugenia Socias, Nadia Fairbairn, Seonaid Nolan, and especially Kora DeBeck for your collaboration and support. I am so lucky to have Ryan McNeil, Andrea Krüsi, Jade Boyd, and Rod Knight in my corner; you have been enormously generous colleagues and dear friends from the beginning. Thank you also to my staff, students, and trainees for your careful engagement with and support of this work over the years, in particular Cathy Chabot, Madison Thulien, Reith Charlesworth, Dan Manson, Trevor Goodyear, Cameron Eekhoudt, and Monique Sandhu. Essential administrative support was provided by Carly Hoy as well as past and present staff at the BCCSU's At-Risk Youth Study field office. Last but certainly not least, since 2018 I have had the honor of working with a fierce and fabulous group of young people who make up my research team's youth advisory council. Thank you for each and every insight and argument, and for keeping me accountable to what matters most.

This project was supported by salary awards and research grants provided by UBC, Canadian Institutes of Health Research, U.S. National Institutes of Health,

Michael Smith Health Research BC, Vancouver Foundation, SickKids Foundation, Frayme, and Making the Shift. Ethical approval for various components was provided by the Providence Health Care–University of British Columbia Research Ethics Board. Part III is a revised version of Danya Fast and David Cunningham, "'We Don't Belong There': New Geographies of Homelessness, Addiction, and Social Control in Vancouver's Inner City," *City & Society* 30, no. 2 (2018): 237–262. Part IV is a revised version of Danya Fast, "Going Nowhere: Ambivalence about Drug Treatment during an Overdose Public Health Emergency in Vancouver," *Medical Anthropology Quarterly* 35, no. 2 (2021): 209–225.

This book would not have been possible without my family. After our daughter Anna was born in 2019 and throughout the COVID-19 pandemic, my partner, Bari, stayed home with her so that I could spend my days writing and running a research program. My parents, Gina and Jerry, provided additional countless hours of child care. Of course, their logistical and emotional support began long before 2019, encompassing my many years as a student and then a postdoc and new faculty member at UBC. Thank you Bari, Anna, Gina, and Jerry for making life such a joy even while writing about increasingly devastating subject matter.

When I started writing this book it was not about those who lived and died young in Vancouver as a result of an unprecedented toxic drug supply. Never could any of us have imagined the unthinkable loss of life that was barreling toward us as the first several years of this project unfolded. Now we live braced for the next phone call, the next email, the next message telling us that someone else is gone. To those we have lost far too soon: we remember you, and we miss you. This book is for you.

DRAMATIS PERSONAE

Lee

Lee was twenty-two when I met him in 2008. He was a member of the Cree First Nation and spent the earliest years of his life on a reserve in Alberta before moving through various group homes in that province. In 2006 he relocated to Vancouver, where he moved frequently between stays in different shelters, privately owned SROs, and supportive housing buildings across the time I knew him.

Lee died as a result of a violent incident in East Vancouver in late 2014.

Lula and Jeff

Lula was eighteen and Jeff nineteen when we met in 2009. Lula is Kaska Dena First Nations but left the place where she was born when only a few days old, following her adoption by a loving family in Vancouver. Jeff is originally from Toronto. Lula and Jeff have two children together, and Lula had a third child in 2017. Lula's second pregnancy allowed her to secure more stable housing in Wenonah House (a women-only supportive housing building) from 2012 to 2017. Over the years I knew him, Jeff lived in the Mackenzie Hotel and the Lakeshore Hotel, before moving into the Greystone Hotel in 2016. He and Lula both lived at the Greystone from 2017 to 2021.

Jordan

Jordan was eighteen when he first arrived in Vancouver after hitchhiking across the country from Ontario. He and I met in 2008, when he was twenty-three. Unlike most of the other young people I knew, Jordan lived in the Downtown Eastside neighborhood across the entire time I knew him. He was well known in that neighborhood, although he regularly considered trying to leave it.

Jordan died from an overdose in his room at the Beachwood Hotel in 2016.

Nancy

Nancy was nineteen when we spent time together at the Trafalgar Hotel throughout 2010. Nancy moved back to Montréal in 2011.

Janet and Johnny

Janet had just turned twenty-one when I met her in 2008. She was born in a small town in Ontario but grew up in Vancouver. Janet stayed at the Lighthouse shelter in 2008 and lived at the Trafalgar Hotel from 2009 to 2010. Janet adamantly refused to move into supportive housing downtown. In 2010, she took off to Port Coquitlam and didn't spend significant periods in downtown Vancouver again for nine years. Over the majority of the time we knew each other, Janet camped outside with her on-again, off-again boyfriend Johnny in various spots located across the suburbs of Greater Vancouver.

Rayna and the Lost Boys

Rayna was nineteen when I met her and several other members of the Lost Boys (including Janet) in 2008. She grew up in the Downtown Eastside and remained in the downtown core over the course of our acquaintance, although rarely staying in any one place for long. Rayna occasionally reflected on her positionality as a "white-looking" Indigenous young person in the city, expressing confusion about how her Indigeneity shaped—or could shape—where and how she belonged in the city and, possibly, elsewhere.

Rayna died from an overdose in 2011.

Carly and Connor

Carly was nineteen and Connor twenty when I first met them in 2008 at the Lighthouse shelter. They have two children together, and Carly had a third child in 2016. Carly and Connor avoided moving into supportive housing in downtown Vancouver across most of the time I knew them, instead moving between periods of homelessness and market rental housing. Eventually, Connor moved into Northwest Apartments, where he lived from 2016 to 2020.

Carly died from an overdose in 2018.

Patty and Joe

I met Patty and Joe in early 2008, shortly after Patty arrived back in Vancouver again after traveling home to Edmonton. Patty was nineteen, Joe twenty. They both came to Vancouver from Alberta, but Joe is originally from Saskatchewan. Joe is Cree First Nations. Patty identified herself as Indigenous during a number of our conversations over the years. Patty and Joe stayed at the Lighthouse shelter in 2008 and 2009. After it was shut down, they were moved into the Trafalgar Hotel. Patty also lived in the Mackenzie Hotel, and Patty and Joe lived at the Lakeshore Hotel and St. Mary's. Joe lived in the Greystone Hotel from 2015 to 2019.

Patty died from an overdose in her room at the Lakeshore Hotel in 2019.

Shae/Trix

Shae was nineteen when I first met them in 2008. They came to Vancouver from Alberta after a time of significant family and mental health crisis that included a period of involuntary institutionalization. This experience haunted Shae as they moved across various institutional settings in Vancouver. From 2008 to 2014, Shae lived in the Lighthouse shelter, the Mackenzie Hotel, Northwest Apartments, and Arbutus House, before moving into market rental housing in 2015.

When I knew them, Shae was a vocal member of the gay community, performing drag under the name Trix. Over time it became clear to Shae that Trix was more than a drag persona, and they began grappling with whether they were a trans woman.

Aaron

I met Aaron in 2008 when he was nineteen. He had just arrived in Vancouver and eventually stayed at the Lighthouse shelter. Aaron is a member of the Kwanlin Dün First Nation and grew up in different group homes in Whitehorse, where, as he grew older, he also regularly spent time with aunties, uncles, and cousins. Many of his family members also made their way to Vancouver over the years. After the Lighthouse shelter shut down, Aaron was moved into the Trafalgar Hotel. He also lived in St. Mary's and Northwest Apartments. By 2017, Aaron was spending all of his time in the Beachwood Hotel, where his best friend lived.

Laurie

I met Laurie in 2008 when she was twenty. She was staying with her new boyfriend, Aaron, at the Lighthouse shelter. Laurie identified herself as Indigenous during a number of our conversations over the years. Like Aaron, she grew up cycling through multiple foster care and group homes, interspersed with periods of running away to live on the streets and with her biological parents in East Vancouver. Across the years I knew her, Laurie lived at the Trafalgar Hotel and St. Mary's, although she spent most of her time away from these places and long stretches of time sleeping outside. In 2016, Laurie and Aaron broke up, and soon after Laurie began dating Kevin, whom she quickly began referring to as her husband.

Terry

I met Terry in 2008, when he was nineteen. Terry identified as Indigenous. He remained close with his adoptive grandmother as he cycled between group and foster care homes as an adolescent and spent numerous periods of time in juvenile detention and jail. He longed to reconnect with the other members of his adoptive family. During the years I knew him, Terry spent many years living outside and staying at shelters. During 2014 and 2015, he lived in St. Mary's.

Terry died from an overdose in 2020.

Shane

I met Shane at Passages (a youth detoxification and treatment site) in 2017 when he was nineteen. We kept in touch over the course of that year as he moved from Passages to Horizons (a longer-term treatment center) to a second-stage recovery house.

Jessica

I met Jessica at Horizons in 2018 when she was sixteen. We kept in touch over the course of that year as she completed a six-month program at Horizons and transitioned into youth-dedicated supportive housing and independent living through government support.

Raymond

Raymond was nineteen when I met him at a youth safe house in Greater Vancouver in 2017. He is Anishinaabe First Nations and moved from Winnipeg to Vancouver when he was fourteen to reconnect with an uncle who was living in the Downtown Eastside. When we met, Raymond had recently aged out of government care and been released from jail. He was moving between short stints in safe houses and periods of street-based homelessness.

Rachel and Gordo

Rachel was twenty and Gordo nineteen when I first met them in 2018. During that year they shared a camp in Port Coquitlam with Janet and Johnny.

Laura

Laura was twenty-two when I met with her a couple of times in the field office in 2017.

Laura died from an overdose one week after our second conversation.

Dom

Dom was sixteen when I visited with him over a couple of days at BC Children's Hospital.

Dom died from an overdose in 2020.

PLACES

THE FIELD OFFICE

A frontline research office located in the Downtown South of Vancouver where I worked full-time from 2008 to 2009. From 2009 I regularly frequented this office to conduct more formal, audio-recorded interviews with young people and supervise students and staff.

SHELTERS, SINGLE ROOM OCCUPANCY HOTELS (SROS), AND SUPPORTIVE HOUSING SITES

The Lighthouse

Located in the Downtown South of Vancouver, the Lighthouse opened as an emergency cold weather shelter in the winter of 2008 and was frequented by several of the young people I knew. In the summer of 2009 the Lighthouse was shut down amid complaints from neighborhood residents, with the promise that shelter residents would be moved into recently acquired government-owned SROs.

Trafalgar Hotel

A government-owned (but yet-to-be-renovated) SRO in the Downtown South where a number of young people, including Patty and Joe, Laurie and Aaron, and Janet, lived between 2009 and 2010. Many were moved directly into this building after the Lighthouse shelter was shut down.

Mackenzie Hotel

A government-owned SRO in the Downtown South where a number of young people, including Patty, Lee, Shae, and Jeff, lived between 2009 and 2010. It was similar in feel to the Trafalgar, and many were moved directly into this building after the Lighthouse shelter was shut down.

Beachwood Hotel

A privately owned SRO in the Downtown Eastside. Jordan lived here from 2011 to 2016. Aaron began crashing here with his best friend in 2017.

Arbutus House

A supportive housing building for people living with HIV. Shae lived here between 2013 and 2014.

Lakeshore Hotel

A government-owned SRO located on the edge of the Downtown Eastside that was later renovated into supportive housing. Patty, Joe, and Jeff lived here between 2010 and 2020.

St. Mary's

A supportive housing building that included a dedicated floor and programming (YouthNow) for young people living with mental health and addiction issues. A number of those I knew, including Patty and Joe, Laurie and Aaron, and Terry, lived here for periods of time from 2010 to 2020.

Northwest Apartments

A supportive housing building that included a dedicated floor and programming (YouthNow) for young people living with mental health and addiction issues. Aaron and Shae lived here between 2013 and 2014. Connor lived here from 2016 to 2020.

Wenonah House

A supportive housing building for self-identified women, including women with children. Lula lived here from 2012 to 2017.

Greystone Hotel

A supportive housing building located in downtown Vancouver. Joe, Jeff, and Lula lived here between 2015 and 2020.

HOSPITALS

St. Paul's Hospital

Vancouver's large inner-city hospital serving young people ages eighteen and older.

British Columbia Children's Hospital

A large children's hospital providing pediatric care to young people ages eighteen and under.

TREATMENT SETTINGS

Passages

A short-term (typically one to two weeks) residential detoxification and treatment center for young people ages fourteen to twenty-four. The facility was closed by the local health authority in 2022 due to concerns about the safety and efficacy of this "social" or "community" model in the context of an ongoing overdose emergency.

Horizons

A long-term (three to six months) residential treatment and recovery program for adolescents and young adults.

Fern Grove

A long-term (up to one year) residential treatment program for pregnant individuals and new parents.

THE BEST PLACE

INTRODUCTION

This is a book about a group of young people at a particular moment in time. It traces their intimate and institutional trajectories as they contended with poverty, homelessness, addiction, and the colonial past and present.[1] It is also a book about a particular place. Vancouver is internationally celebrated as one of the world's most beautiful, cosmopolitan, and livable cities but is also recognized globally as a ground zero for successive waves of public health emergency.[2] The young people who are the subject of this book were in many ways relegated to the social, spatial, and economic margins of this city. Yet they were also often at the very center of city life and state projects (Henry 2019), including the protection of life in the context of an ongoing and unprecedented drug overdose crisis (Das and Poole 2004).

For over two decades, Vancouver has been significantly transformed by escalating wealth accumulation and rampant gentrification and events like the 2010 Winter Olympic Games (Barnes and Hutton 2009; Blomley 2008; Ley 2012). The city has also been remade by public health emergencies, from HIV/AIDS in the 1990s to the COVID-19 pandemic. These states of emergency have intersected with an entrenched affordable housing crisis and growing problems of visible homelessness and addiction. What has unfolded in Vancouver informs visions of the creative, sustainable, and multicultural city globally, as well as national and international discussions about progressive drug and housing policy and harm reduction. The policies, strategies, frameworks, guidelines, and interventions generated in this setting and the province of British Columbia (BC; where Vancouver is located) often go on to be emulated across Canada, North America, and elsewhere.

In this book I explore these politics of place from the perspectives of urban poor young people who use drugs. I demonstrate that my interlocutors engaged with and embodied these politics in ways that exceeded the assumptions of many policy makers, practitioners, and academics. Their senses of place could include a fragile sense of belonging and being at the center of *something* rife with potential in "The Best Place on Earth"—a promotional slogan that for a time appeared in government advertising for the province of BC, including on license plates commemorating the 2010 Vancouver Olympics. They could also include deep fears that one was somehow getting lost or going nowhere in a setting of entrenched poverty and deprivation.

Previous anthropological work has skillfully examined the experiential and therapeutic trajectories of addiction (Raikhel and Garriott 2013a) and how these intertwine to constitute drug use as a lived experience and object of intervention (Hansen 2018; Knight 2015). Anthropologists have demonstrated the importance of "following" (Meyers 2013; Raikhel and Garriott 2013b) people, therapies, and ideas about addiction across time and place to reveal some of the effects of dispossession, industrial decline, criminalization, and white supremacy (Bourgois and Schonberg 2009; Garcia 2010; Knight 2015; López 2020; Netherland and Hansen 2016; Pine 2019; Sue 2019). This work has deftly illuminated the suffering generated by political, economic, and historical processes as well as the forms of resistance and resilience enabled by injury, grief, and rage (López, Abbey-Bey, and Spellman 2018; Ralph 2014, 2017).

Drawing on fifteen years of fieldwork in Greater Vancouver, I build on and diverge from this previous work by attending to the more ambivalent forms of life that were emerging among some young people who use drugs in Vancouver, where particular dreams of place knocked up against a frenetic pace of public health intervention and urban change to continually remake possibilities and the trajectories of substance use and care. These forms of life did not always coalesce around suffering or political action, or the prescriptions of even the most progressive policy makers, providers, and activists. Rather, they coalesced around particular kinds of affective intensities and rhythms (Million 2013; Stewart 2007) and the moves, escapes, "flights" (Deleuze 2006), and forms of suspension that they animated (Biehl and Locke 2017a).[3] Following Tanana Athabascan scholar Dian Million (2013, 46), for some Indigenous young people the colonial past and present could itself take the form of a "felt, affective relationship" that was sensed but not always spoken, particularly in ways that fit neatly with medicalized imaginaries of risk, harm, substance use "disorders," and treatment.

Rather than anchoring my analysis with concepts like structural violence, governmentality, or biopower or adopting lenses of resilience or resistance, I trace the multiple, shifting, and highly affective senses of place and broader forms of life that emerged among those I followed, as they moved across places that included run-down shelters and single room occupancy hotels (SROs), supportive housing buildings, and residential drug treatment and recovery facilities.[4] Previous anthropological work has examined how affects like melancholy, uncertainty, and grief shape forms of life in communities marked by drug use, violence, and loss (Garcia 2010; Ralph 2017; Stevenson 2014). Ethnographies of addiction and treatment have explored affect as one of the materials out of which experiences are made (Garcia 2010; Knight 2015; Meyers 2013; Schüll 2012), and several scholars have signaled the importance of attending to senses of eventfulness (Cohen 2001) and boredom (German and Latkin 2012; Jervis, Spicer, and Manson 2003; Mains 2012; Masquelier 2019; O'Neill 2014). However, anthropologists have not yet adequately probed the affective rhythms and intensities that are released by public health emergencies and interventions and what these do as they move through and accumulate in bodies, substances, pharmacotherapies, and places that include both care settings and the various "elsewheres" (Meyers 2013) through which addiction and therapy travel.

Here, I explore how the "weighted and reeling present" of addiction and care in Vancouver can be productively explored through what Kathleen Stewart (2007, 1) calls ordinary affects: those visceral, surging forces that animate bodies, places, things, encounters, and atmospheres and constitute a "felt knowledge" (Million 2013, 67) of a situation and its possibilities. The rhythms and intensities that I describe came into view in bodily gestures, such as when young people paced excitedly around the living room in a residential treatment center, talking rapidly about their plans for when they got out, or when they slumped down tiredly in that same living room, mumbling that they were completely worn out. They surfaced in forms of sociality, such as the frenetic fun of intensive drug use, and became legible in strategies and their failures, including the decision to go to treatment again (and again). They circulated in dreams and expectations, such as the feeling that this time, with the help of housing or opioid agonist therapy, things were going to be different, or the impression that programs and services got them nowhere. While affect is often characterized as prediscursive (Massumi 2002), it seemed to me that young people did attempt to put a palpable sense of stagnation into words when they used the language of boredom and phrases like "getting lost" and "going nowhere" in the city. Alternatively, they evoked a sense of momentum when they used the language of business and described feeling like they were "in *something*" rife with potential.

Vancouver is home to one of the most well-developed public health and "poverty management" (DeVerteuil 2003) infrastructures in North America, in terms of both services and research capacity (Murray 2011; Roe 2009/2010). The city's care assemblage—to borrow a term from anthropologist Andrea López (2020)—has long centered on the downtown core and in particular the Downtown Eastside neighborhood, where a plethora of services offer shelter, food, health care, harm reduction, advocacy, and religious salvation to those in need. Vancouver's Downtown Eastside continues to be imagined by many as the "proper" destination of the visibly homeless, addicted, and mentally ill in the city (Liu and Blomley 2013; Woolford 2001). On the corner of Main and Hastings streets, in the heart of the Downtown Eastside, the open drug market operates 24/7. Street-level dealers sell crack cocaine (crack), miscellaneous opioids, and crystal methamphetamine (meth), while others try to make a few bucks by "flipping" (selling) their prescription methadone and hydromorphone. Those who are buying dart in and out of alleyways bustling with activity. Others camp out along sidewalks, congregating on lawn chairs or sheltering under tents, tarps, and multiple propped-up umbrellas, often surrounded by possessions and variously procured merchandise (some purchased, some shoplifted, some traded) carefully laid out on the concrete for resale. The Downtown Eastside is also inhabited by a large number of people who do not use drugs at all. Many are simply poor. On Pender Street, just one block south of Hastings, elderly people can be seen walking along Chinatown's vibrant streets, socializing and shopping. Some occasionally dig through public garbage bins for discarded cans and bottles (known as binning), which can be redeemed for a small cash refund. The neighborhood is also a racialized space (Razack 2007); many of its inhabitants are Indigenous. These demographics reflect the continued presence of Indigenous people on land owned and occupied by Coast Salish peoples for at least ten thousand years and the disproportionate burden of social suffering carried by Indigenous people in Canada (Anderson 2013). In this book I foreground ongoing Indigenous space- and place-making in and beyond the Downtown Eastside, contributing to scholarship on settler-colonial and Indigenous urbanism that seeks to reveal the continued dispossession and displacement of Indigenous people in cities while simultaneously contesting totalizing narratives that define Indigeneity and urbanism only in relation to colonialism (Dorries 2023; Dorries et al. 2019; Peters and Anderson 2013).[5]

Property values have been steadily rising in the Downtown Eastside, and it has been significantly transformed by gentrification in recent years. It is now edged by two of the city's most desirable neighborhoods. To the east, Strathcona's charming heritage homes are increasingly inhabited by socially progressive, upwardly mobile young professionals. To the west, Gastown's historical buildings have been converted into exposed brick office spaces, trendy restaurants, and high-end furniture shops. Even in the heart of the Downtown Eastside, new condominium developments, fashionable eateries, and hipster coffee shops intermingle with the few remaining well-worn storefronts and bars, SROs, and buildings of various nonprofit organizations, creating what some might characterize as a sort of "poverty chic."

The care assemblage in downtown Vancouver expanded rapidly with the HIV/AIDS public health emergency of the 1990s. During the decade and a half that followed, various protocols, action plans, and agreements identified street-based homelessness, addiction, disease, and hunger as problems that could be better managed through partnerships between government, local businesses, nonprofit organizations, researchers, and others. The Vancouver Agreement, which came into effect in 2000 and ended in 2010 (the year of the Winter Olympic Games), was a particularly high-profile attempt to coordinate alliances between various state and nonstate actors; by 2009, the agreement resulted in more than seventy inner-city projects funded through almost fifty different organizations (Murray 2011; Vancouver Agreement 2010). The expanded infrastructure that emerged out of these protocols, action plans, and agreements has supported things like widespread needle distribution and accessible methadone, heroin maintenance trials, and, notably, North America's first supervised injection facility (known as Insite).

These biopolitical interventions stabilized the HIV epidemic, and this success story has been incorporated into the city's mythology. Vancouver is home to world-class public health and harm reduction services and programs and regarded as a model for other places beset by similar problems (McCann 2008). However, over the same period, street-based homelessness and the concentration of visible poverty and addiction in the downtown core persisted. This "second generation" of Vancouver's public health emergency is still often framed today through the language of "mental health and addictions" (Boyd and Kerr 2016; Vancouver Coastal Health Authority 2023a). Most recently, an unprecedented drug toxicity and overdose crisis has claimed the lives of over ten thousand people in the province of BC since an official public health emergency was declared in 2016, including over two thousand young people between the ages of ten and thirty (BC Coroners Service 2022). As a result, harm reduction services and sites have increased and the city is actively expanding a more coordinated system of substance use treatment for people who use drugs, with a particular focus on adolescents and young adults under the age of twenty-five (Government of BC 2019). The churn of intervention that largely began with the HIV/AIDS emergency continues into the present with the COVID-19 pandemic, heat domes, and other climate change-related crises.

In this book, I trace aspects of this institutional story by bringing into view the trajectories of one group of young people who use drugs, a population that has received comparatively less attention in Vancouver and other urban settings. Those who are addicted to drugs in the context of unstable housing and homelessness in Vancouver are largely defined through their relationships with the Downtown Eastside and another neighborhood I call the Downtown South, where the majority of "street youth" services are located. The Downtown South is within walking or biking distance of the Downtown Eastside, and young people often move between the two neighborhoods, sometimes several times a day. While technically a part of the Downtown district, the Downtown South goes largely unnamed. If it is called anything at all, it is usually lumped in with the adjacent West End neighborhood, which extends down to Vancouver's popular tourist beaches on the western edge of the downtown core and across to the large, forested area of Stanley Park and surrounding Seawall in the northwest corner of the city center—another of Vancouver's most popular attractions for locals and foreigners alike. Stimulant and opioid use are commonplace in the Downtown South, but in contrast to the Downtown Eastside, the buying and selling of drugs occur mostly out of public sight. Busy shopping malls, nightclubs, bars, and upscale condos are interspersed with a handful of shelters, nonprofit service hubs, SROs, and government-owned supportive housing buildings, to an extent disguising the marginality that exists there.

The Downtown Eastside and Downtown South were powerful organizing symbols in the lives of those I followed (Fast et al. 2009). Many regularly frequented the street youth and "drug user" services located there. But as we will see, they often refused these conceptual and geographic boundaries, traveling frequently or relocating completely to the suburbs of Surrey, Port Coquitlam, New Westminster, Burnaby, and beyond. Acts of memory, dreaming, desire, and return integrated Vancouver's inner-city and suburban drug scenes with still other places that transcended these places in space and time (Anderson 2013; Gordillo 2004; Massey 1994). In this book, one of my goals is to write against the idea of isolated, inner-city drug scenes, instead bringing into view young people's more expansive dreams of place and geographies in and beyond the city (Ralph 2014).[6] Another is to uphold their drive to singularize out of populations and categories such as street youth and drug user (Amit and Dyck 2006; Biehl 2005). I take seriously Unangax̂ scholar Eve Tuck's (2009) challenge to move away from damage-centered research that further pathologizes young people, especially Indigenous young people, and toward work that attends closely to their desires for things to be otherwise (Biehl and Locke 2017b). I describe a group of individuals who mostly actively refused to inhabit the "suffering slot" (Robbins 2013), including as a source of resilience and resistance within a transforming urban landscape that was producing new forms of stagnation, dislocation, disappearance, and loss. Nor were my interlocutors always content to inhabit the forms of life idealized by harm reduction policies and programs. They articulated much more widely shared dreams of place in Vancouver, which many believed really *was* one of the best places on earth. These dreams included nine-to-five jobs and exciting careers, engaging in leisure activities in the evenings and on weekends, and making a home and creating a family with a romantic soulmate and beloved pets. Young people often insisted on their inclusion in these kinds of urban imaginaries and asserted a powerful sense of belonging in the city, even as they contended with entrenched poverty, addiction, (re)institutionalization, illness, and injury. Vibrant forms of life emerged to continually exceed policy framings that would position them as the mere victims of structural violence and settler colonialism or as unfortunate problems to be solved (Dorries 2023).

Those I followed are part of an urban population for whom everyday living has indeed been rendered problematic in similar ways by structural forms of oppression. On the streets of Greater Vancouver, they navigated the everyday emergencies (Bourgois and Schonberg 2009) of poverty, homelessness, and unstable housing; addictions to crack, heroin, fentanyl, meth, and alcohol; blood-borne infections, overdoses, mental health crises, and cycles of voluntary and involuntary institutionalization; and volatile drug deals, sex work transactions, and romantic relationships. In the places of their childhoods and on the streets (in some cases, one and the same), the overwhelming majority grew up in circumstances of severe poverty and routinized physical and psychological crises that included frequent assaults but also the everyday violence of perpetual uncertainty and dislocation. More than half were apprehended from their birth families by the state and subsequently grew up cycling between multiple government foster care and group homes before aging out of the system at nineteen and then again at twenty-five (depending on the mandates of different programs and services—some supported adolescents up to eighteen, and others supported young adults up to twenty-four). Almost all had spent time in psychiatric wards, juvenile detention centers, and jail, and only a small number had graduated from high school. They were also marred by the structural violence of historical and political economic forces ranging from over a decade of austerity politics in the province of BC (Van Veen, Teghtsoonian, and Morrow 2019) to the continued effects of settler colonialism in Canada and the global war on drugs. In what follows, I acknowledge the everyday emergencies and continuum of violence (Scheper-Hughes and Bourgois 2003) that all of the young people I followed were forced to navigate. But I also stay close to their dreams and desires and the "not yet" and "not anymore" moments in their stories-so-far (Tuck 2009, 417).

This book weaves together ethnography and creative nonfiction. I have employed a number of literary devices in order to both protect young people's confidentiality and evoke their complex personhoods (Gordon 2008), perspectives, and trajectories. While none of the dialogue is fabricated, it is not verbatim transcription. I have edited dialogue to align with how I experienced their words and sentiments and so that it more concisely moves forward the stories that my interlocutors and I talked about telling over the years. I have also changed dates and locations when these could be matched with official records and allow the various professionals in young people's lives to possibly identify them. With the exception of two hospitals, all of the names appearing in this book are pseudonyms, including those of shelters, SROs, supportive housing sites, treatment facilities, and programs, to retain what anonymity is possible. However, anyone familiar with the service landscape of Vancouver's inner city may be able to identify some of these places. While these kinds of localities are important to the arguments I make, my observations extend beyond the specific places I describe. Finally, despite the critiques I develop, I want to acknowledge at the outset the tremendously challenging and lifesaving work done by those on the front lines of Vancouver's poverty management and public health infrastructures. Like their young "clients," these providers are struggling to navigate the complex realities of urban change and a near constant state of public health emergency in a city where funding is increasingly tied to policy agendas.

This book is divided into five parts made up of many short chapters. It is structured as a roughly chronological account of the transformation of Vancouver's inner city and outlying suburban drug scenes and care assemblage. It also unfolds through deeply personal relationships between myself and a relatively small number of young people. My research over the past fifteen years has involved hundreds of individuals. Here I tell the stories of only a few, whom I followed for periods ranging from five years to over a decade. I trace their stories as they move from the streets into an emergency cold weather shelter and then into run-down SROs, supportive housing facilities, and drug treatment and recovery settings. We follow them into the various elsewheres and everywheres to which they routinely escaped. The book also jumps around in time to evoke complex senses of place and self in the city and how these intersected with young people's trajectories and emerging forms of life. In the second half of the book I introduce a few other individuals whom I encountered for much shorter periods—from a few days to a few weeks or months—weaving these briefer encounters together with my longer-term ethnography. I recognize that focusing on a small number of individuals itself constitutes a form of disappearance. So many people and stories are missing from the pages that follow.

While the sections and chapters are designed to build upon one another conceptually to contribute to anthropological discussions of place, addiction, affect, and intervention, the structure of the book is intended to suggest the impossibility of tidy theorizations that allow us to draw easy conclusions about these young lives and the programs and services designed to help them. Instead, a juxtaposition of stories, voices, encounters, and images attunes us to an affective churn (Fast 2021) of addiction, intervention, and urban change in Vancouver, and how it alternatingly propelled young people forward or held them still as they attempted to make a place and home for themselves. I am trying here to evoke the partial and unfinished (Biehl and Locke 2017b; Tuck 2009) nature of their stories and my relationships with them as well as moments when stories and relationships were suddenly and irrevocably ruptured. I provide "only contour lines" around experiences, encounters, and affects (Meyers 2013, 118). As Todd Meyers (2013, 5) describes in his ethnography of adolescents enrolled in addiction treatment in Baltimore, I had to contend with different kinds of "shadows and disappearances" among those I followed. As we will see, there were many ways that young people could disappear from this project, including their deaths.

Some of the shadows I encountered were shaped by my positionality. There were lines of flight and forms of refusal (Simpson 2014) that I could not—or knew that I should not—follow. I am a white settler who has spent fifteen years working closely with Indigenous young people who use drugs. I tell the stories of a small number of those individuals here. I have attempted to write these stories with great care (Garcia 2010), working closely with these individuals whenever possible to make decisions about what has and has not ended up in this book. I have tried to write in moments of refusal (Simpson 2014), while honoring others by writing nothing at all. None of this resolves crucial questions about the extent to which I am speaking for Indigenous young people in this book, "mining" their words and experiences for my own scholarship (Todd 2019). I must sit with this lack of resolution, allowing readers to judge for themselves the balance of care and harm that this book achieves.

Questions of speaking for go beyond Indigenous young people. I grew up in the place that is now known as Vancouver, in circumstances of tremendous privilege. I do not have lived experience of entrenched poverty, homelessness and unstable housing, and intensive drug use. I did not come to this project with a background in drug user and antipoverty activism or service provision within Vancouver's care assemblage. My interlocutors and I therefore occupied very different positions along axes of race and class. Most of the time, we inhabited very different urban geographies. This shaped the kinds of stories young people told me and how they told them. It shaped what came into view and what remained in shadow, obscured from me. But I would be remiss if I emphasized only the differences between us. There was commonality, too—or desired commonality. And there were the ways in which my positionality shifted across time.

When this project began, I was in my mid-twenties and therefore close in age to many of those I followed. Over time, I entered and completed graduate school and transitioned into a role as a faculty member at the University of British Columbia. Across the fifteen years of this project, I was attempting to apprehend the social, spatial, and affective worlds created by the rapid implementation and scale up of various interventions aimed at adolescents and young adults and increasingly contributing to their animation. By 2017 my research was carried out via large team grants and partnerships with a group of healthcare providers, program managers, policy makers, epidemiologists, and young drug user activists, whose collective goal was to improve the delivery of a continuum of substance use care and fight for change. We were all of us implicated in the "will to intervene" (Lorway 2021) to save the lives of young people who use drugs in Greater Vancouver and shared a crushing sense of futility (Brodwin 2011) when we were unable to do so. In 2019 I, like so many of those I followed, became a mom.

Thus, this project involved different kinds of proximity and distance between researcher and researched. Interestingly, rather than emphasizing the social, economic, geographical, and political distance between us, young people would often steer the conversation toward our proximity. For example, they often pointed out how our itineraries in the city overlapped—even if it was the case that they regularly took the bus up to the University of British Columbia to shoplift, while I was attending graduate school there. Moreover, in certain moments this project seemed to create desired forms of social and geographical proximity for them—proximity to imaginaries of a "normal" life in the city that I sometimes reflected back at them and to the "nice places" they longed to inhabit. In addition to allow-ing us to develop friendships across large differences in positionality (see also Culhane 2011), our research encounters brought young people into a number of spaces that it would have been difficult for them to access under other circum-stances. We frequently shared meals and cups of coffee at what they referred to as nice coffee shops and restaurants. These opportunities to sit indoors as regular paying customers were a stark contrast to the humiliation of attempting to sneak into fast-food restaurants several times a day to use the bathroom or seek refuge from the rain, only to be kicked out a short time later. We also went on many day trips together, traveling in my car to photograph the suburbs of their childhoods, popular tourist attractions like Vancouver's North Shore Mountains, and the neighborhoods where they imagined living in the future. During these outings, even the toughest self-proclaimed gangsters gleefully played around with my iPhone, checking Facebook and carefully crafting playlists for our car ride.

In these very same moments, I could become a mirror of the worst kind for young people. At times they became painfully aware of the differences between us—differences that, as Dara Culhane (2003/2004, 97) notes, "stretch[ed] back into historical time, permeat[ed] the present moment, and shape[d] the future." I had an apartment, an iPhone, and a car. I had a university education and a "real job" doing research. These were things that they deeply desired and wanted to believe that they would one day attain once they had "pulled their lives together." The fact that I had them and they did not could generate anger, sadness, and resentment. Ultimately, I was "accessing the lines of social mobility from which they [were] removed" (Culhane 2011, 260).

Over time, some young people positioned themselves within this project as fellow researchers rather than research subjects, even though I officially began employing community-based participatory action methods only in 2018 (Thu-lien et al. 2022). Long before that, however, on more than one occasion they made a point of showing me books that they had checked out of the public library on the history of the "drug problem" in Vancouver and offered up insights gained from their reading in this and other related areas, such as the 2008 global economic recession (see also Robertson 2006). Over the years, many began referring to this project as "our university project," and more than once I over-heard someone explaining on the phone that they had to hang up now because they had a job working for the university. In certain moments, I became an employer. In others, I was an advocate or simply someone who could help them during moments of crisis. Young people rarely conflated my role in their lives with that of various service providers; the latter were overwhelmingly viewed as individuals who had significant control over some aspect of their lives, which I did not. However, they did regularly ask me for help, and during many of these moments of crisis they made it clear that what was happening was not a part of our research. These were encounters that should be left in shadow.

Most of those I followed did not want me to draw easy lines between us—me as an urban citizen who belonged within Vancouver's beauty and promise, and them as "at-risk youth" relegated to the social, spatial, and economic margins. My goal, therefore, is not to contribute to broad generalizations about the situation of street youth or young people who use drugs in Vancouver or elsewhere, although I do build on previous work that demonstrates how tracing individual patterns of experience can be productive for making and unmaking what is known about a collectivity and collective problems (Biehl 2005; Garcia 2008). I have also been purposely reserved in my use of theory. While I find certain concepts useful for thinking about how processes of urban change produce new forms of life and harm for young people (as I largely elaborate in endnotes), I agree with others that too much reliance on theory can "foreclose the possibility of letting things be vulnerable and uncertain" (Garcia 2010, 35). It can eclipse young people's own intelligences and theorizations. Here, I stay close to their words and "arts of living" (Biehl 2013, 583). This book is for them, and for those who loved and cared for them—and love and care for them still—as much as it is for fellow anthropologists and academics.

PART 1

DREAMS OF PLACE

LEE, THE BEST PLACE ON EARTH, 2009

"My very first night here—all the lights on Granville Street [in the Downtown South]—it felt like I was in Vegas," Lee said in 2009. "Well—I've never been to Vegas before, right? But, I don't know—it's how I imagine it—from TV and stuff. This is the best, uh, place on earth, I think. Just like the license plates say. It's just awesome out here."

All across the city, in shelters and SROs, beneath overhangs and in doorways, and in public parks and beaches, big-city dreams burned bright amid troubling nightmares.

JEFF, PARADISE, 2009

"I had dreams of Vancouver my whole life before I came here," Jeff said to me the first time we met. It was the spring of 2009. We were standing in an alleyway, leaning against the wall of the Lighthouse shelter. The light was slowly draining from the early evening sky, but the atmosphere was charged, anticipatory. Groups of young people formed and disbanded as they darted in and out of the shelter and up and down the alley. The party was just getting started.

Jeff continued, "It was a recurring, vivid dream of Vancouver as, like, a paradise. I felt like I was at home in the dream. I was walking down Granville Street [in the Downtown South], and there was grass instead of pavement. And I thought to myself, how cool, how awesome it was here. And everything was perfect right until the end of the dream. A tsunami hit me. That's when I got killed and I woke up screaming every time."

BIG-CITY DREAMS

In the public imagination, young people who use drugs in the context of homelessness and unstable housing are often defined through their relationships to place. In Vancouver, they are viewed as out of place when in too close proximity to the city's towering, glassy high-rises and condominiums, expensive bars, restaurants, and shops, and carefully restored heritage homes. In the colonial imagination, Indigenous young people continue to be positioned as out of place in cities full stop, despite long histories of territoriality in these places and continued vibrant presence (Dorries et al. 2019; Peters and Anderson 2013). Yet, young people who use drugs, including Indigenous young people, may be understood as in place on the streets and in SROs and supportive housing buildings in Vancouver's Downtown Eastside and Downtown South neighborhoods, even as gentrification in these neighborhoods increasingly brings them into proximity with homes and businesses from which they are excluded. Alternatively, they may be understood as simply placeless, with nowhere to go.

I began this project expecting to learn how young people made a place for themselves in the social, spatial, and economic margins of the city, and particularly the Downtown South and Downtown Eastside. Yet I was repeatedly confronted with dreams of place that exploded these conceptual and geographic boundaries. As I got to know them, my interlocutors didn't often want to talk about life in the margins, including where they were coming from and where they were currently located. They wanted to talk about Vancouver as one of the best places on earth and to imagine where they were going next.

Vancouver is a hyper-researched setting of poverty and addiction. This project was just one of many that young people could engage with in return for cash honoraria and other material and immaterial benefits.[1] This setting perhaps brought into sharp relief how my research subjects often actively played with damage-centered (Tuck 2009) and suffering slot (Robbins 2013) narratives, at times articulating familiar narratives of risk, harm, and marginality, at others forcefully rejecting them. They could be highly tactical in their use of designations like at-risk youth to gain resources and advantages from sympathetic social workers, judges, researchers, and other professionals. Simultaneously, those I knew were generally not willing to imagine a sense of place or self rooted in the idea of a local street youth or drug user community (Fast et al. 2013) or shared forms of biosociality (Nguyen 2010; Petryna 2002). Nor, in most moments, could these young people be characterized as "righteous dopefiends" (Bourgois and Schonberg 2009) or "urban outcasts" (Wacquant 2008). Instead, they embraced, and felt embraced by, big-city dreams and told many of the same stories of belonging and becoming (Biehl and Locke 2017a; Deleuze 1995) that are, to a certain extent, inhabited by us all (Comaroff and Comaroff 2000; Robertson 2006; Sterk 1999).[2]

LULA AND JEFF, PARADISE, 2012

Over the years that I knew Jeff, I never heard him say anything that contradicted the idea of Vancouver as a paradise. I also never heard him say anything about how his circumstances in the city might reflect the end of his dream, when it became a nightmare. In mid-2012, his perpetually on-again, off-again girlfriend Lula saw things much differently. She was alternating between crashing with Jeff in his miniscule room at the dilapidated Lakeshore Hotel (a government-owned SRO) and sleeping in shelters—or staying up all night, high on meth, to avoid both.

Lula is Kaska Dena First Nations. She left the place where she was born when she was only a few days old, following her adoption by a loving, white family. She grew up in the city and spent her childhood and adolescence living in an affluent Vancouver neighborhood. She recalled often her many childhood vacations, the pop concerts that she went to as a teenager, and the fancy clothes, shoes, and purses she had once owned. Whenever Lula compared her current circumstances to her past, she tended to emphasize all of the ways in which she was now living in a nightmare. This drove Jeff crazy; they frequently fought about their sense of place in the city when we were together.

"Is Vancouver a paradise?" I asked them in 2012 as we sat together in a room at the field office. I had been looking back on that first conversation with Jeff in 2009. By 2012, the pair had been dating for three years. They had one child together, a girl, born in 2011 but not in their custody.

"The Downtown Eastside is obviously *not* a paradise," Lula answered quickly. "Sunset Beach [in the West End], or, you know, the view of the city from Grouse Mountain [on the North Shore], yeah, it's a paradise," she qualified. "If you're living that kind of life where you can go and actually enjoy those places. Which was me, uh, at one point—"

"—If you're a drug addict it kinda *is* a paradise though—the Downtown Eastside," Jeff interrupted sharply. "You don't understand, Lula; in other cities you can't use drugs openly at all. You'll get beat up for using drugs like what happens here." Jeff was originally from Toronto and spent much of his adolescence there involved in low-level, loosely gang-connected crime. In Toronto as in Vancouver, moral worlds of the gang were animated by regular incidences of violence, including to prohibit "out-of-control" substance use while engaging in drug dealing and crime (Fast, Shoveller, and Kerr 2017). "Vancouver is very accepting of drug use. Just look at all the services, and Insite [the supervised injection facility] or whatever, right?"

Lula did not appreciate Jeff's lecturing tone. Annoyed, she clarified, "Yeah, well, there's also a lot of hurt and suffering down there, in the Eastside. And anger and hatred. On people's faces. Including my own."

"But Lula, um, from an overall, *worldwide* perspective, Vancouver is—at least they're not starving to death, and they're not as desperate as, say, in Ethiopia or, um, South Africa," Jeff shot back. His voice was rising as he became increasingly angry about where this conversation was headed. Meanwhile, Lula was getting increasingly angry about how Jeff was speaking to her. I couldn't get a word in edgewise.

Jeff continued, "I've been to South Africa, during the Nelson Mandela election. My uncle worked for CIDA [Canadian International Development Agency]. In other cities people are actually *at war*—there's a war going on in the Middle East right now. That's why I find Vancouver to be a paradise. When you look at it compared to, um, Kabul?"

I tried to steer the conversation to acknowledge Lula's perspective, while also acknowledging Jeff. "Some people say that, here in Vancouver, there is a 'war on the poor' going on. And there is a 'war on drugs.' What do you think about that?" I asked.

Lula opened her mouth to answer, but Jeff was quicker. "*Are* people that poor here though?" he replied. "I could be considered poor, I think? Here. But I don't think of things that way. I find Vancouver a very beautiful and friendly and accepting city. Even in the Eastside, you have a nice view of the mountains."

"Where do you two mostly spend time these days?" I asked, trying to change the subject. Lula's annoyance with Jeff was palpable, and I imagined she might leave at any moment.

"Mostly we spend time close to home, pretty much," Lula answered, laughing nervously. "I mean, Jeff's room there [in the Lakeshore Hotel]. We do a lot of walking around outside, I'd say. Um, go into a lot of Tim Hortons [a local fast-food restaurant] bathrooms. Half an hour later, we come out—'You can't come back!'" She stood up suddenly and imitated the staff kicking them out for injecting meth in the bathroom. Lula and I laughed, but Jeff was livid.

"Lula has to point out all the negative things," he practically shouted. "'Don't come back!' Like we're so *unwanted* and scrutinized here. It's not true *at all*. We're welcome in most places we go to, Lula. And these days, yes, we're mostly in the Eastside, but is that a general question, or just like, nowadays? Because, actually, I'm really new to the Eastside. To the city basically—well five years is not *that* new, but I never really liked to hang around the Eastside before recently. When I got housing there, right? But in general, I'm pretty—I like to travel and go to new places and do new things. I mean, like, my dad's in the military so I moved around a lot as a kid. Like I said, I've been to Africa and stuff. So."

Jeff paused to compose himself. "Lula's making us out to be, like, *rejected* in society. She has a biased view, cause she's from here. And I don't like how Lula does that. Cause it's *not true*. And like, that matters—it means a lot to me. Cause it's my—I love Vancouver. I love it here. I don't ever want to leave."

Lula decided to stop talking. A few minutes later, she abruptly got up and left the room. We left the conversation at that.

SENSES OF PLACE

Places are intersections of histories, structures, memories, imaginaries, and affects. They are always in process, always in motion. Over the past two decades,

Vancouver's urban landscape has transformed. High-priced real estate developments, shops, and restaurants increasingly intermingle with SROs and nonprofit-operated supportive housing buildings and service hubs, some dilapidated, some brand new. This transformation has brought into focus the very different kinds of belonging and becoming that are available to young people in the city (Cahill 2007; Davila 2003; Mirabal 2009). However, among those I followed, the transforming city was incorporated into equally shifting processes of subjective experimentation, resulting in multiple and oftentimes contradictory senses of place and self. By senses of place, I am referring to how the city was remembered, imagined, desired, narrated, and lived, that is, a way of "knowing, experiencing, and relating to the world" (Coulthard 2010, 79).

Crucially, young people's senses of place were formed in tension with other places and geographical relocations and dislocations, which transcended Vancouver and its drug scenes in space and time and could even extend across generations (Garcia 2010; Gordillo 2004; Massey 1994). Entanglements of place and subjectivity were continually made and remade through acts of remembering, dreaming, imagining, and, occasionally, return. Most of those I knew came or fled to downtown Vancouver from elsewhere—other cities, towns, and First Nations reserves (almost always referred to as "the Rez").[3] In relation to these places, the city was generally framed as the site of new and desirable opportunities for work, leisure, fun, homemaking and family making (Henry 2019; Robertson 2007). Ongoing poverty—and in some cases connections to friends and family members already living in the city—meant that many quickly found themselves in neighborhoods like the Downtown Eastside and Downtown South. Yet young people constantly described their plans for creating a "real home" in one of Vancouver's "nice" neighborhoods—not just the Downtown Eastside; getting a university or college education—not just their GED; and going shopping in "normal" stores—not just standing in lines for free food and donations. They spoke about how wonderful it was to live near the ocean and the mountains (even though most had never visited Vancouver's North Shore Mountains until I took them there) and described with pride Vancouver's much celebrated multiculturalism.

LEE, WORLD CITY, 2009

During a conversation in early 2009, I asked Lee if he ever considered returning to the reserve in Alberta where he was born. By his own admission, Lee had been having a hard time in Vancouver since arriving in 2006, although he was working hard to "turn things around." He had recently gotten off crack and stopped drinking, largely through daily, intensive cannabis use and the occasional use of meth (Fast et al. 2014; Paul et al. 2020). However, his living situation was tremendously precarious as he cycled between various shelters, "the worst" privately and government-owned SROs, and periods of street-based homelessness.

"Back home, on the Rez, it's really poor," he said thoughtfully. We were sitting together on a park bench in the Downtown South. Lee's memories of the Rez seemed quite blurred. He had been removed from his family home by the government when he was very young.

"I think [the Rez] is a very peaceful place. Just being in nature and everything, right? But people just sit around all day, cause there're no stores—there's no work there, really. All you gotta do is raise up your kids and go to school. Grow old and be there." After a pause, Lee continued. "Nothing's happening out there. And, um, I don't see myself ever going back—backwards. In Vancouver, though, you have so many different kinds of people, going to work, going shopping, doing this and that—you know what I mean? There's so much to do here, different ways to progress yourself."

Lee became increasingly animated as he imagined the details: "Here, eventually you'll have a good job. You know, get up, take a shower. Go to work. Then take a lunch break—all those kinda things, right? You'll come home from work every day and feel like you did a good job. And you're *happy* because you've got that paycheck every two weeks in a bank account. You're there for two and a half years, and then your salary goes up. I would love to just have *my own house*, right? And have a dog, right? One or two kids—you know what I'm saying? And to be able to do things for your kids—just to be able to go camping on the weekend, or go skiing if you wanted—you know what I mean? Just the *normality* of life. I'm gonna have all that, eventually, when I get my own job and stuff—soon, right? I wanna have—I wanna have—"

"A white picket fence life?" I interrupted, laughing. It was a phrase I had been surprised to hear another young person use the day before, in the context of a similar conversation. "You know that saying? Where you have the perfect family home and it has a white fence around it?"

"Yes," Lee answered matter-of-factly, refusing to laugh along. "I want that. Here. I'm looking for work right now—restaurant work, landscaping. But it just seems like there's nothing."

Almost two years later, Lee's living situation remained highly unstable, and he continued to move in and out of intensive crack, meth, and alcohol use. We met up just one week before the opening ceremonies of the 2010 Winter Olympic Games in Vancouver to review some photographs he had taken related to an arts-based project that we were developing (Fast 2017).

Leading up to the 2010 Games, a small number of the young people I knew expressed strong resistance to them, in ways that aligned with the throngs of protesters demanding "Homes, not Games!" for urban residents experiencing homelessness and unstable housing. They vowed to meticulously document how various, long-circulating rumors were being realized as the Games drew nearer—how people who were visibly poor and addicted were being arrested for petty infractions such as jaywalking so that they could eventually be jailed for failing to pay fines, for example, or how they were being relocated to the suburbs and herded into government-owned SROs in downtown Vancouver so that they were out of sight when the athletes and tourists arrived.

Most of those I knew, however, told me about how much they were looking forward to the Olympics. As an Indigenous young person and, as he put it, "one of the true, original Canadians," Lee said that he felt included within Vancouver's much celebrated multiculturalism, which was particularly on display during the Games. Rather than highlighting their social, spatial, and economic exclusion, for Lee and a number of others the Games created space for desired forms of belonging.

"I'm excited for hockey, snowboarding, downhill skiing, even bobsled!" Lee said that day in 2010, as we sat together in a Blendz coffee shop on the corner of Broadway and Commercial Street in East Vancouver, a bustling transportation hub where young people often congregated to meet up, "hook up," drink coffee, and deal drugs. In 2010, this particular Blendz was often jokingly referred to as "the band office" because of the large number of Indigenous people of all ages who lived in the surrounding area and regularly congregated there to socialize.

"I'm going to have a good time and just really *enjoy it*," Lee continued, as we watched a group of teenagers taking turns to bang noisily in and out of the front door of the coffee shop whenever they saw someone they knew approaching. It was pouring rain, and the front windows were foggy with condensation. Outside, a young girl wearing pajama pants and slippers was huddled beneath the overhang, panhandling. The teenagers mostly ignored her even as she loudly appealed to passersby for spare change and cigarettes, which many were intermittently smoking. They were jumpy with excitement, engaged in an intimate choreography of greetings, loud conversations, and hushed asides. Their jackets and purses were strewn across numerous laminate tables and plastic-coated chairs. I had seen many of them in this Blendz on previous occasions. This was their place.

Lee seemed relatively unfazed by the commotion. "They delivered a new TV to the shelter, so I'll be able to watch it *all*," he said. "And, I'm excited to walk around the city—my home, you know?—with so many other people from all over the world, you know? And to go on that big zip line they put up [between two buildings downtown]."

A group of Elders entered the Blendz. Once they were seated with their coffees Lee halted our conversation so that he could go over and greet them. When he returned, he told me that he knew them from events at the Aboriginal Friendship Center, located a short bus ride away. He said that he had been trying to reconnect with his culture more lately. "One of those guys had an Olympics ID," he said, beaming. "He got a job doing security work. Wow! It means he gets to ride the bus for free until the Games, and then while they are on, too. And he heard a rumor that McDonald's [fast food] might be *free* for athletes and staff for the whole two weeks [of the Games]! Man, I wish I could get something like that. But it's too late now, I guess."

Lee cycled through government foster care and group homes throughout his childhood and in the winter of 2010 was living in a particularly notorious privately owned SRO in the Downtown Eastside. He frequently opted to stay outside or in shelters rather than deal with bed bugs, constant noise, and regular violence in his building. He was critical of the chronic instability that had characterized his childhood and aware of how it extended into his present. More than once he had tried with difficulty to put this into words for me.

"When I was young, and, like, taken from my family—" he began once, and then paused. "Living on the Rez is really hard when you're a kid," he finally continued. "It's very hard. Especially if your family can't take care of you because of drug issues, drinking, or whatever it is." He paused again. "I mean, it's very rare for a Native family to be together. If you know what I mean? And then it's almost like jail, when the government is controlling your life, and they would move you and move you until you were eighteen. Against their will. It gets to a kid, very much."

Eventually, he added, "When I was a kid, I wanted to be with my family more than anything else. But they [the government]—they were pushing me in different directions and, uh—everything, uh, kind of *explodes* and doesn't come back together and—" he trailed off. "It's not like a magnet, right?" he said after a while. "And now you want to try and recover—by working on yourself, but—" he trailed off and did not elaborate further.

Given Lee's past and present and how both seemed to be weighing on his future, we might expect that he would be among those shouting "Homes, Not Games!" at local protests. After all, many would argue that the Games made much spectacle of Indigenous inclusion while diverting millions of dollars that could have been used to improve the material conditions of urban Indigenous young people like Lee. However, in conversations in 2009 and 2010, Lee consistently embraced the Olympics. The photographs that he showed me that day in 2010 were not focused on his marginality; over the course of what became a five-year photo essay project, he would be steadfast in his refusal to take images of where he lived and slept. Rather, most images captured the comfortable future and progress he imagined for himself in the city: going to work, playing sports on the weekends and in the evenings, and living in what he referred to as his dream place. He would take these kinds of photographs recurrently. In 2012, for example, I was struck by the numerous images he had taken of various construction sites. I initially assumed that he was developing a political commentary on processes of gentrification. But instead Lee pointed out small details in the photographs and explained that he planned to get a job in construction doing a particular kind of welding once he had recovered from intensive substance use.

Did Lee "misrecognize" his entrenched marginalization and exclusion while others actively resisted it? I don't think so. Instead, I follow others (Mahmood 2005) in cautioning that we need to be wary of creating a politically prescriptive dichotomy between resistance as agency and conformity as subordination. Such an understanding imposes a teleology of progressive politics on analytics of place, power, and desire—a teleology that makes it hard for us to see and understand senses of place and self among those occupying margins that are not necessarily encapsulated by narratives of resistance.

WHERE I'M GOING, LEE, 2011

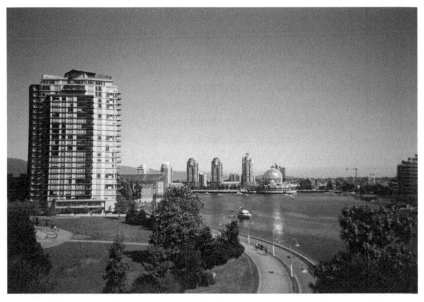

JORDAN, NORMAL PLACES, 2012

It looked like it was going to rain as I waited outside the entrance to the Beachwood Hotel in the Downtown Eastside. Jordan rarely invited me into his building, which he referred to as a "shithole." The SRO where he had been living for the past year had a nondescript, anonymous feel. The hotel entrance was an unmarked black door, the reception area where guests had to be signed in and out by a building attendant not visible from the street. On either side of the entrance there were now a couple of fashionable café bars; inside, a half dozen smartly dressed young people had their Mac laptops open in front of them. An older man with a disheveled appearance and noncoherent speech was sitting in his wheelchair in front of one of the café entrances, shaking an empty McDonald's coffee cup. Those who walked by largely ignored his requests for change.

The block that Jordan lived on was changing rapidly. In addition to the new café bars, across the street an older building had recently been knocked down. An advertisement for new condos was tacked up on the temporary yellow fencing around the construction site. The new development was called "The Flats," a reference to a sort of trendy internationalism that perhaps particularly resonated with those who have spent time living and traveling abroad. The photograph that accompanied the text was of an interracial couple holding hands and smiling as they walked through the neighborhood. It celebrated the kind of multiculturalism and eclecticism that the revitalized Downtown Eastside neighborhood—and the City of Vancouver itself—was imagined to embody.

Jordan told me many times that he dreamed of getting a "real" place in the Downtown South—"a nice little bachelor apartment close to the ocean" was how he once put it. To make that happen, Jordan first had to get a "real, nine-to-five job." In one of the most expensive housing markets in the world, his meager monthly welfare checks would be inadequate to cover the monthly rent plus an initial damage deposit.

"I've never actually, to this day, ever had a real job," Jordan admitted to me on a previous occasion. "Well, I've had one actual job—at the Old Spaghetti Factory [chain restaurant] in Calgary, Alberta. I worked there for three and a half months. It was the greatest time of my life," he sighed happily. Jordan hitchhiked across Canada when he was eighteen; Calgary was his last stop before Vancouver. Once in Vancouver, he often talked about how his addiction to heroin "completely took over," and he had been unable to secure work since.

When Jordan finally emerged from his hotel that day, he informed me that there was a community garden he wanted to show me. This represented a departure from our usual itineraries. We rarely strayed more than a few blocks from his hotel and the handful of services in the Downtown Eastside that he frequented on a daily basis. As we walked east toward the garden, Jordan told me that he was several days "clean" off opiates.[4] He had been enrolled in a heroin maintenance trial but decided to quit, even though rumor had it that the waiting list for the trial was hundreds of people long. "I was one of the first people they asked to be in it," I remembered him saying several months before, sounding pleased.

Jordan was well known in the Downtown Eastside. For several years he had been directly involved in the politics of place that surrounds the neighborhood. This politics takes various forms, including world-leading harm reduction initiatives like North America's first supervised injection facility (known as Insite), yearly marches to remember the neighborhood's missing and murdered women, and squats and tent cities to protest gentrification. Jordan had even appeared in a documentary about harm reduction in the Downtown Eastside. He had often bragged about this, but as we approached the entrance to the community garden he told me that he was furious about the outcome of his participation in the film. That was the thing about Jordan: he could refuse his place in the Downtown Eastside and the subject position of a service-dependent young drug user in certain moments—and articulate an explicitly politicized subjectivity in relation to the neighborhood, drug use, and services like Insite in others.

"[In the documentary] they used footage of me and put my name under it and everything without my permission," he said angrily, vigorously smoking a cigarette. "They *outed* me as a *drug addict*." I had asked him why he decided to leave the heroin maintenance trial. In his mind, the connection between the two events was obvious. "[The people who are running the trial are] just *giving* you drugs. Turning you into a junkie. You think I want to be stuck in these programs for the rest of my life? No. It's a revolving door. They say they're trying to help you but they're not really helping you because I don't *want* to be a drug addict. I *care* what society sees me as. I don't go to food lines—I don't go to *any* shit like that. I buy my own food at a normal store. I actually really only go to Insite just to say hi to people. I know all the staff there," he added quickly, smiling.

Jordan continued, "I don't want to be labeled as a junkie down here who's going nowhere. I can't handle the fact that, someday, somebody might say to my daughter, 'Hey your dad was down here shooting up, blah, blah, blah.' 'Your dad's a junkie.' You know, say I'm walking through the mall with my daughter, trying to buy her a birthday present, her first outfit for school—" he trailed off. Jordan seemed to be imagining what it would be like to do something like that—to go to a mall without being asked to leave by security, to have the extra money to buy gifts for his daughter, or to have any kind of relationship with his daughter, who was nearly three years old. He had told me many times that he longed to be a real dad to his two children. "You know what I'm saying?" he continued finally. "And then to have her hear, 'Hey, your daddy's a junkie' from someone who saw me down here?" He shook his head.

Walking through the community garden, Jordan talked about how much he loved "normal" things like flowers, gardening, and being in nature. We wound our way along a wood chip pathway through neatly divided plots. Jordan greeted and attempted to strike up a conversation with the few people we saw who had decided to brave the weather and work on their garden plots. He snapped some photographs with my camera. These would be a stark contrast to the other images he had taken in the weeks prior, which focused on the most degraded features of urban space—the run-down alleyways, concrete alcoves, and empty lots where he had slept and used drugs before getting a room in an SRO—and details like discarded syringes and human feces. The world he captured on camera seemed polarized between beauty and filth. Jordan later articulated that the photo essay he was working on was about what is visible on the surface of an internationally celebrated city like Vancouver and what is hidden from public view and visible only to "people like him." Through his photo essay, Jordan seemed to be positioning himself as a part of both landscapes.

"I haven't always been like this—I've spent a year clean here, too. And I loved it," Jordan emphasized that day in the garden. "I love Vancouver. There's so much to see and do here." He picked up a discarded syringe out of the foliage and held onto it for proper disposal. We emerged from the community garden onto an open lot. It used to be a place where people congregated and camped in tents but was now vacant and scattered with idle bulldozers, in the process of being redeveloped into some kind of training facility. The elevated tracks of the SkyTrain transportation line—connecting downtown Vancouver with the city's outlying suburbs—loomed overhead in the distance. Jordan attempted to get a few photographs of the open lot with a passing train in the background. A man in a dirty sports jersey and jeans darted out of a narrow path along a chain link fence to our right and ran past us. We walked along the same path littered with old beer cans, takeout containers, and other garbage and came out where a recycling depot is located. There were several older binners (individuals who collect recycling for a small cash refund) out front, unloading carts full of used cans and bottles. This was not a future Jordan imagined for himself.

"I'm a college boy," he said confidently as we walked past the recycling depot. "I studied culinary arts. Computer sciences and shit like that—I loved it." Jordan had been incarcerated for most of his adolescence and completed some college-level courses in prison. "Yeah, I'm a quarterback," he boasted. "I was one of the best in Kingston [Ontario] when I was a kid. I'm *still* a good athlete. I still rollerblade along the Seawall all summer long." He looked at me, possibly wondering if I was going to question his continual reframing of the facts of his childhood and sense of place in Vancouver. Certainly, his descriptions of rollerblading all summer long and playing on sports teams as a child diverged from his frequent lamentations about the fact that he "never left" the Downtown Eastside and had "never so much as been taken to a baseball game as a kid." What interested me, however, was how remembered and imagined geographies continually shaped the entanglements of place and subjectivity that he was contending with. These wider geographies alternatingly positioned him as unambiguously out of and in place in the Downtown Eastside.

"I came out here for the surf, and for the chicks," Jordan reminisced as we walked back toward his SRO. "I've always wanted to go to Wreck Beach out by UBC [the University of British Columbia]. That's one place I would really like to go. But yeah." He sighed. "I want to get my life together. I want to go to university. I never went to a *real* school. I wish I could've. I'd like to do what *you do* honestly—teach people about health and stuff. Or be a police officer. All my life I wanted to be a police officer. I get really intimidated when I'm around normal crowds though," he said nervously, lighting another cigarette. "Like, in a way I find you really intimidating. Just the little things you say—like when you told me how expensive this camera is." He adjusted the strap I always insisted he keep around his neck so that there would be no chance of him dropping my camera, and looked away.

DANYA AND NANCY, THE FIELD, 2010

Of course I had my own dreams of place in Vancouver. As I began undertaking research for my PhD in late 2010, these dreams included imaginings of what a more immersive period of fieldwork would look like. As an undergraduate anthropology student I was captivated by the ethnographies assigned by my various professors and their own tales from the field, many viscerally depicting suffering and affliction. I was awestruck by the long-term and intimate encounters out of which such renderings emerged. The kinds of physical and emotional proximity bound up in these encounters were striking and seemed to reflect deep individual and disciplinary desires to bear witness to, understand, document, and help others. Now of course I recognize that desires for these forms of proximity also reflect deep-seated colonial impulses and disciplinary anxieties around what constitutes authentic anthropological fieldwork. Underlying many of the stories my professors told and the ethnographies they assigned was a now thoroughly problematized imperative to get closer—as close as possible, perhaps—to the margins and the marginalized through immersive fieldwork (Pels 1999; Shuman 2006).

As a master's student I followed in the footsteps of my teachers. For a time I too lived and undertook research in a densely populated, sprawling urban settlement under the hot sun of the tropics. These footsteps, particularly when taken by a white woman, were being increasingly troubled within the discipline of anthropology, but I did not yet have enough awareness and language to reckon with that. I would soon be taken to task and forced to reckon with my positionality in the field, not by anthropology and its critics but by many of the young people whom I would come to work with over the next decade and a half in Vancouver. I would also quickly learn that positionality is not solely the concern of the anthropologist (Fast 2016). Our research subjects may be equally concerned with how to position themselves in relation to researchers and research studies. They, too, are engaged in navigating the forms of proximity and distance that are embedded in anthropological encounters across time. This is perhaps particularly the case in hyper-researched settings like Vancouver.

My doctoral research focused on the city in which I was born and had lived for most of my life. However, like my master's research, it was not a departure from what was in vogue in anthropology at the time it began. Homelessness, addiction, and "street cultures" have long captured the discipline's imagination, and so-called suffering subjects stand at the center of much of our work (Robbins 2013). Philippe Bourgois and Jeff Schonberg's photo-ethnography of the Edgewater homeless, *Righteous Dopefiend*, was published in 2009, the same year I entered a PhD program. At this time, Vancouver's inner-city drug scenes had long been zones of intense research, surveillance, and monitoring, where people who used drugs on the streets were subjected to the gaze of a steady stream of anthropologists, epidemiologists, public health experts, police officers, providers, workers, activists, artists, politicians, and the media (Culhane 2005). I joined this procession of observers and interlocutors as an anthropologist doing research at home, in settings that were both highly familiar and foreign to me.

In order to document the intimate lifeworlds of those who use drugs in the margins, anthropologists have slept on the streets and in homeless camps and spent countless hours in SROs; we have exposed ourselves to police harassment and arrest and been in hospital rooms as those we have developed close relationships with—friendships, in many cases—are treated for life-threatening overdoses, infections, and mental health crises (Bourgois 1996; Bourgois and Schonberg 2009; Knight 2015). When I began a more concentrated period of fieldwork for my PhD at the beginning of 2011, I imagined that it would look similar to all of this. And in many moments over the years it has. But it has also diverged significantly from these familiar tropes.

My doctoral research was broadly focused on how young people understood, experienced, and navigated their place in a rapidly transforming city in the context of addiction and entrenched social, spatial, and economic marginalization. I had been working as a qualitative interviewer and then coordinator for a large, university-affiliated urban health research center since late 2007; when I began intensive fieldwork for my PhD in 2011 I had already developed close relationships with approximately twenty-five young people. It seemed imperative that I now immerse myself in these individual's worlds to an even greater extent. I felt the personal and disciplinary need, the desire, to get even closer to their everyday lives—perhaps, I imagined, by finding work in one of the government-owned but yet-to-be-renovated SROs that many inhabited by 2011 or by spending more prolonged periods with them in the tent cities that frequently sprung up across Greater Vancouver both in protest to and as a temporary solution for the housing crisis. But as I began initiating conversations with young people about the kind of research I hoped to do, many made it clear to me that they had their own, competing desires for what our research encounters might look like.

"So, what do you want to do right now?" Nancy asked in 2010 as she furiously smoked a cigarette. "I'm bored." We had been hanging out in her room at the Trafalgar Hotel for a few hours, drinking coffee, smoking cigarettes, and chatting. There didn't seem to be much more to catch up on, and I was getting bored too.

My time at the Trafalgar was often punctuated with updates: this person owed that person money but had taken off somewhere; this couple was fighting about this and that couple was fighting about that; and could I go and talk to so-and-so about that thing that had happened yesterday so that they didn't try and beat up so-and-so over a misunderstanding? Young people banged endlessly through the hallways and in and out of each other's rooms, often seeming to stoke the fire of the latest drama rather than working to extinguish it. But that day it was noticeably quiet. Everyone was broke and waiting for Welfare Day in two days' time, when they would receive their monthly social assistance checks.

"Um, I don't want to do anything," I replied, suddenly awkward. "I mean, just this, I guess? I mean, what would you be doing if I wasn't here?" I asked.

"I would probably just be sitting around in here, like we are," Nancy said. "I'm tired today." She laughed quickly, as she did almost every time she paused between sentences. This constant laughter seemed less out of amusement than some sort of discomfort. Nancy continued, "And every once and a while I would go down to see my buddy [and meth dealer] on the second floor. Wait around for my stupid boyfriend to come back, because he's flailed off [taken off while high] somewhere, again. Maybe go out and look for him eventually, I guess? And that's about it." She changed her tone and asked more provocatively, "Why do *you* want to be here so badly, anyways?"

"I guess, uh, I want to get a better sense of your everyday life," I replied, sensing that my answer would not land easily with her and might piss her off. "Uh, what it's like to live here—uh, in this building, but I guess, like, in this neighborhood too, and just in this city as a whole?" Nancy stared at me, seemingly skeptical. I tried a different approach: "I mean, some people who do the kind of research I do, they actually move into places like this, or work in places like this, so that they can really get a sense—"

She cut me off, almost angrily "—that is the *stupidest* thing I've ever heard. First of all, if you worked here, I would freaking *hate* you. I'm not trying to be mean, but I would *hate* you. We all hate all the managers. They are goofs who think they're better than us."

She became increasingly worked up. I could no longer tell if she was talking about me, her manager, or both of us: "Like, don't treat me like I'm an *idiot drug addict*. I'm not. I'm a *normal* person. I've lived in *normal* apartments, in a house and shit, when I was little. I know how to cook. Like—I know how to clean. I know how to go to school and I know how to work a normal, like, job. I used to work in a fast-food restaurant, before my mom died. Like, this isn't how I live—normally."

"Okay," I replied carefully. "I hear you. I get what you're saying. But I'm still curious—what do you think about the other part—about a researcher actually living and sleeping in a place like this? Because the idea is that most of the research down here is all surveys in an office—there aren't many researchers who actually, uh, spend time with people in these places. And that could be good—"

"I think it's *stupid*, and it kind of makes me mad," Nancy replied without hesitation. She continued forcefully, "Like—this place, okay? This place is not who I am. Like, my boyfriend and I are actually thinking about, like, moving in together, to an apartment in Surrey. A normal freaking apartment with a kitchen and bathroom and all that shit. When I move there, you can come over, and we can hang out for as long as you like and have our little 'chats' there—" she did that quick laugh again "—because that will be, like, a home, and feel comfortable, and all that, right? That's why, actually—I actually prefer that, like, we hang out at a coffee shop, or even in your car—in *normal places*—because that's actually where I am more comfortable. Like, I'm not comfortable in this shithole room, in this shithole hotel. That's why I keep my room like this." She gestured to the mess that surrounded us. "That's why I keep getting kicked out of these places. It's not me. It's not me. Like—I'm not like that."

Research subjects are often astute analysts who have developed clear ideas about how "we"—students, health and social science researchers, and various professionals—position "them" (Culhane 2011), and those I followed were no exception. They often pushed against my personal and disciplinary desire for particular kinds of closeness—for example, a closeness premised on spending time together in what young people often framed as "shithole," "junkie," "crackhead," and "drug addict" spaces. They didn't always want me around, but not for the reasons I was worried about when I first started talking to them about my desire to spend time in the places where they lived out their everyday lives. They didn't necessarily view my presence in these places as an invasion of their privacy—by 2011 I had long been accompanying many of them as an advocate to appointments with social workers, housing workers, welfare workers, probation officers, methadone doctors, and officials from the Ministry of Children and Family Development (often referred to as simply "the ministry"). Nor did it seem to be a question of establishing more of what we sometimes refer to as rapport. Rather, they didn't want to identify themselves or be identified with certain kinds of places in the context of my project—a project that they knew perfectly well could further slot them into categories such as at-risk, addicted, and marginalized.

So, rather than spending a lot of time together in what they framed as drug user spaces, many I came to know forcefully suggested that we spend time together in what they often referred to as normal places. These included coffee shops, fast-food restaurants, public gardens, beaches and parks, my car, and, as they often put it, the real homes that they still had access to belonging to a select few family members and friends. They spent much of our time together forcefully rejecting the claims made for and about them by many health and social science researchers, including claims about who they were (members of a street youth or drug user community, for example), who they were not (normal young people pursuing work, leisure, and homemaking in one of the world's most livable cities), and where and how they belonged in Vancouver (as street youth, drug users, and social service clients confined to the inner city, for example, versus urban citizens whose geographies included nicer neighborhoods and spaces). Their desires to redraw the lines between "us" (those who unambiguously belonged within the city's beauty and promise) and "them" (those positioned in the margins) and to singularize out of categories like street youth and drug user shaped the boundaries they placed around their participation in this project. This was evident in the stories they told me, but also in the conversations they sometimes refused to have (those premised on their expertise as urban poor drug users, for example). It was evident in the places they insisted we go to and photograph together, such as community gardens, public beaches, and Vancouver's North Shore Mountains, but also in the places they refused to spend time in and photograph together.

Even as they actively used and sold drugs on the streets, lived in SROs and supportive housing buildings, and regularly accessed various key nodes in downtown Vancouver's care assemblage, distancing themselves from particular kinds of drug user spaces and drug using others seemed to be an important way of aligning themselves with their dreams of place in the city. They also often distanced themselves from long-term involvement in my research.

LEE, NOT THESE SERVICE PLACES, 2009

"Can I get in touch with you again?" I asked Lee as we walked back to the field office together beneath the bright lights of Granville Street.

His response was immediate: "Actually, I was thinking about finishing my [high] school this year, right? All I got is another year. Go to college or something. I'm still young and I wanna pursue certain dreams, right? I'm gonna get a place and I'm gonna get a job here really soon, so I probably won't be around these service places here all that much."[5]

JORDAN, NORMAL PEOPLE, 2008

"You're gonna go home now, and I'm gonna stick in the back of your head," Jordan turned to me and said as he was leaving the field office in 2008. "Because I'm mostly not a 'drug person.' I know normal people here in all different parts of the city. People with expensive houses, with cars and gold. Even in the Downtown Eastside now, there are people like that. My friends look just like you."

FRICTIONS

In a very different setting, Anna Tsing (2005) uses the concept of frictions to make sense of a social drama of the Indonesian rainforest, where unpredictable, oftentimes fraught encounters—between New Order army officers and nature lovers, university students, and village elders, for example—nevertheless provided an opening for collective action. I saw how young people's desires infused many of our research encounters in unexpected ways. As we came to know each other, they were no doubt well aware of the social, economic, and geographical distances between us. And yet they often used our research encounters as opportunities not to underscore our differences but rather to align themselves with what they framed as normal forms of belonging and becoming in the city. They insisted—sometimes quite angrily, sometimes with great sadness— that they weren't like the other people they imagined were a part of my research and asserted that we were much more alike than I—a researcher who was perhaps trying to help or save at-risk youth—had considered. In some of these moments—especially toward the beginning of this project—our disparate desires and imaginings of what we were doing together crashed up against each other, producing awkwardness and sometimes even conflict.

As others have noted (Castañeda 2005; Elliott 2014; Elliott et al. 2015), paying close attention to these kinds of moments of misunderstanding, miscommunication, and friction across vast differences in power and privilege can provide an opening for carefully thinking through, oftentimes together with our research subjects, what is at stake in a particular time and place.[6] In this project, what seemed to be at stake for many of those I followed included the imperative of survival in the context of the everyday emergencies of poverty, violence, pain, and trauma, but also the dreams, imaginaries, moralities, and configurations of care, love, and possibility that animated everyday life. What was at stake was the need to shake loose from determinants and definitions like crackhead and junkie, "drunken Indian" and "white trash"—but also "IDU" (injection drug user), "NFA" (no fixed address), and "SUD" (substance use disorder)—even as many daily inhabited these labels to access services, support, and research honoraria or to get a break from a sympathetic judge, worker, or police officer. Many of those I came to know had been trying to distance themselves from these kinds of labels and "policy-relevant codes" for their entire lives (Robertson 2006, 302). Immersed in Vancouver's hyper-researched inner-city drug scenes, they quickly realized that they also had to push against well-worn social science scripts— about community and resilience in the margins, for example (Fast et al. 2013)— to assert desired senses of place in the city. This was also what was at stake for them as they enrolled in yet another study about at-risk youth in downtown Vancouver in order to make ends meet, but also, perhaps, to position themselves in the city in particular ways.

DANYA, AROUND DOWNTOWN, 2008

This research began in a small field office near Granville Street in the Downtown South, where I worked full-time as a qualitative interviewer and then research coordinator from late 2007 to the fall of 2009, when I began my PhD. From the outside, the field office was barely distinguishable from the legal practice beside it, providing a degree of anonymity for those who went in and out. Each time the door to the office opened, a mechanical voice that was part of the alarm system repeated "Front door," "Front door," followed immediately by a ding-ding-ding sound once the door was closed again. Inside, rows of chairs were lined up against the walls to create a waiting area. There was a tired-looking coffee machine in one corner and a battered dresser full of donated clothes and toiletries in another. In the back of the room was a desk with an aging computer, used by office staff to track participation in a large epidemiological cohort study of youth who use drugs (other than or in addition to cannabis) in the context of street involvement, defined as being homeless or without stable housing and regularly accessing street youth services. On the walls were posters demonstrating various safer drug cooking procedures and one that showed the steps for safer injecting through a series of anonymous photographs. By 2012 some of the photography that young people had produced for my own project was up on the walls, and a short time later a flat-screen TV was installed. Thick soundproof doors and curtained windows separated two interview rooms from the chaos of the adjacent hallway, through which participants trudged back and forth to use the washroom and see the cohort study nurse. The presence of a nurse, donated clothes and toiletries, and free coffee and food meant that many young people did not distinguish this research setting from "other service places" in the neighborhood, although they rarely conflated my role in their lives with that of a service provider. During the first few years of my research, we would often sit in one of the two interview rooms at a sterile laminate table, facing each other with an audio recorder between us. A single lamp provided dim, unobtrusive lighting. While we spoke, some individuals would obsessively arrange and rearrange the contents of their backpacks. Others would pull out coloring books and markers, usually shoplifted from local drug stores and supermarkets, or ask for paper and a pen so that they could draw. Some put their heads in their arms on the table to rest.

This research also began in a particular shelter in the Downtown South. In 2008 most of those I knew referred to themselves as homeless. Some were sleeping outside, in public parks, on beaches, and beneath overhangs and bridges located across and beyond the downtown core. Others were couch surfing or squatting at friends' places or cycling from shelter to shelter. In winter 2008, many began staying at a temporary emergency cold-weather shelter opened in the Downtown South. At the Lighthouse shelter, I first got to know many of those whose stories fill these pages, including Lula and Jeff, Carly and Connor, Patty and Joe, Shae, Terry, and Laurie and Aaron. Carly and Connor were the first to invite me to spend time with them at the Lighthouse after we had gotten to know each other at the field office. I had met these other individuals before as well, and so I found myself able to visit with multiple young people and couples while in and around the shelter.

The Lighthouse was intended to accommodate around forty people during the coldest months of the year; additional government funding allowed the shelter to stay open through the summer months. The extended life of the shelter occurred amid growing objections from nearby condo occupants, who complained about open drug use, fights, and public sex in the shelter's vicinity. In summer 2009, the Lighthouse was officially shut down, with the promise that shelter residents would be moved into recently acquired government-owned SROs. I followed young people as they were moved into various buildings. By 2010, a great deal of my fieldwork was occurring inside these places.

Finally, this research began in and around the Downtown South and Downtown Eastside, even as it quickly became clear that my project would continually escape these boundaries. Shortly after beginning my job as a qualitative interviewer at the field office, I was connected with Kyle, a hired research assistant who described himself as having one foot in and one foot out of downtown Vancouver's drug scenes. Kyle introduced me to the constellation of public, semi-public, and private spaces in which these drug scenes—and so much beyond them—came alive: the streets, alleyways, SROs, shelters, drop-in services, parks, and Vancouver Art Gallery steps where young people met up and broke up, laughed endlessly together and fought fiercely with one another, bought, sold, and used drugs, and made and unmade homes and families with each other in the city. Some of these places I knew from my own adolescence in Vancouver. However, my privileged glimpses into the city's drug scenes were markedly different from the trajectories that led all of those I followed to these places, where they were thrown into new forms of destitution, homelessness, addiction, and crime by recurring forms of personal and institutional experience (Fischer 2003; Garcia 2010). My previous experience with drugs and drug scenes didn't ever seem to matter, regardless. It was Kyle's skillful introductions and guidance that allowed me to start spending time in these places; there, I eventually got to know Lee, Jordan, and Janet and her gang of Lost Boys.

JANET AND THE LOST BOYS, NEVER NEVER LAND, 2008

"Downtown Vancouver is Never Never Land. And *we're* the Lost Boys," Janet said by way of introduction. She clarified that by calling themselves the Lost

Boys, she and her friends were referencing both the story of Peter Pan (Barrie 2004) and the popular 1987 film about a gang of teenage vampires. They were a fierce and disheveled bunch, with haloes of brightly dyed hair and dirt underneath their fingernails. In 2008, they could be seen panhandling along Davie Street in the West End and binning in the back alleys, ferociously protective of their turf. Everyone seemed to know the Lost Boys; they even maintained mostly amicable relationships with some of the local cops ("keep your friends close and your enemies closer," Janet often joked over the years). They hated shelters and were in 2008 avoiding the Downtown Eastside, preferring to camp in Stanley Park and other well-hidden spots located in the West End and Downtown South. They dressed like the punks and nomadic train-hoppers who arrived at Pacific Central Station each summer, but many were originally from or had grown up in Vancouver. Several had pet rats.

"It's good, and it's bad, right?" Janet continued. "This little fantasy world we've, uh, created for ourselves. We get to be kids again, down here. We get to have fun. We don't ever want to grow up, right? Even if it f-cking kills us."

A number of the Lost Boys described themselves as growing up on the streets of downtown Vancouver, with parents who were also "in the life." They had all cycled between government group homes but ran away to their families and the streets again and again. When I met them in 2008 they were spending most of their time in and around downtown Vancouver, moving frequently between its different neighborhoods. They never stayed put for long. Beyond the frenetic fun that often accompanied going on various missions to track down money, stolen merchandise (merch), drugs, and the people who had them, "being everywhere" was a way of keeping themselves safe, avoiding violent and controlling romantic partners and those they owed money to. It was also a means of ameliorating chronic boredom. Downtown Vancouver may have been a fantasy world characterized by fun and blissful suspension, but this world was also regularly punctuated by troubling moments of stagnation. Young people also contended with various forms of dislocation, which they often summarized as a sense of "getting lost" in the city. They could become unmoored by increasingly "out of control" addictions, interpersonal violence, and infections. For many, the inevitability of being lost to these was powerfully embedded in downtown Vancouver, particularly the Downtown Eastside (Fast et al. 2009).

In 2010, Janet found out that she had hepatitis (hep) C during a rare stay in a residential detoxification (detox) center. At that time, things had become so dire in terms of her tumultuous living situation at the Trafalgar Hotel, her abusive relationship with her then-boyfriend, and her declining health that she had finally accepted an offer of help from local outreach workers. She was picked up near where she was doing sex work by an outreach van and driven straight to detox, where standard blood work had revealed that she had hep C. Her diagnosis had so devastated her that she had declined further offers of help, including longer-term treatment, out of a sense that some part of her was irreparably "ruined."

Many of those I followed over the years expressed similar sentiments after being diagnosed with hep C and, in a few cases, HIV. Rayna, another member of the Lost Boys, was matter-of-fact when she described to me in 2008 how she was making sense of the fact that she had been diagnosed with hep C and, recently, HIV. She was nineteen years old.

"My parents grew up down here," she began, as we sat together on the steps of the Vancouver Art Gallery in the pale late afternoon winter sun, only a few feet away from a rowdy congregation of other young people. There was a jumpy excitement in the air as things began to get underway for the evening.

"They're pretty well known in the Downtown Eastside, and they're drug addicts so therefore I watched my parents do it all my life and I started doing drugs when I was, like, ten years old. Whatever." Rayna paused, a look of irritation passing over her face as she watched two of her friends discuss with increasing volume what such-and-such had done earlier and how such-and-such had had every right to have reacted in such-and-such way.

She continued somewhat abruptly. "I thought about trying injecting, and I thought that it was a very bad idea—I knew the risks, right? It's a really hard decision to make. When you're a Downtown Eastsider, either you're going to be a full-on junkie or you're not going to be. You can still maintain some integrity, but—" she trailed off, continuing to follow the drama unfolding beside us. More people had now joined the discussion, which was hovering somewhere between a full-blown argument and a joking exchange.

"Sometimes that's the only option you really have, right?" Rayna said, turning to look at me. "Being a junkie and eventually killing yourself. Once you stick a needle in your arm, you keep sticking a needle in your arm because it's the only thing that makes you feel better. I was in self-destructive mode. I thought, I'm going to eventually get AIDS, and I'm going to eventually die. That's what it's like when you live down there. My biggest problem was that I always *knew* that I was going to go down. So I hit rock bottom. I didn't have any reason to care, which is why I contracted hep C, a couple years ago. And just this past little while, from using a dirty needle, I found out that I'm HIV-positive. It's my fault," Rayna added quickly, even angrily. "That was my choice. Because I knew damn well— pretty much since I was a little kid—you stick a dirty rig [needle] in your arm, it's your f-cking fault if you get HIV."

As she said all of this, I tried to keep my face neutral, to simply sit there listening, rather than jumping in to contradict her with comments like "of course it's not your fault, Rayna!" or "you don't have to die from this" or "you're feeling better about things now, aren't you?" I had said these sorts of things in these kinds of moments in the past; I would do so again on occasion as my research progressed. I couldn't help myself. But by the time this conversation was happening I had been told by enough individuals, including Rayna herself, that platitudes weren't helpful. On another occasion, not long before that conversation on the Art Gallery steps, Rayna had chastised me, researchers, and "service people" in general for assuming that death was the worst thing that could happen to a person. Rayna was talking about her possible death sometime in the not-too-distant future. She was not suicidal but seemed to be feeling the weight of the violence she regularly endured at the hands of romantic partners and sex work dates. On that occasion, I responded by saying something along the lines of "I can't accept that" and offering to help connect her with various services and providers. "I've had way worse things happen to me in my life," she snapped back at me. "I'm not afraid of dying, compared to what I've been through." Could I just listen to what she was telling me?

Sense of place is an embodied knowledge of the world; it delimits a field of workable possibilities in the locations out of which it is formed. For Rayna and various others, a sense that they belonged in a place like the Downtown Eastside powerfully shaped how the past was interpreted and revised ("It's my fault I got HIV"), what futures were possible to imagine ("I was always going to go down"), and how the present moment was perceived and acted upon. While Rayna often felt in place (at times, hopelessly so) in the Downtown Eastside, she occasionally reflected on how she and her family seemed to be perpetually out of place as "white-looking" Indigenous people. As Rayna put it once, "I look white but I know from my family we *aren't* white, right? But, like, I'm unsure of whether I am even *allowed* to say that I'm Native because I look so different from my Native friends down here, right? And that was also my family's experience, too, before we came here, right? Kind of not being *allowed* to be a part of that."

For Rayna and the other Lost Boys, it could be particularly difficult to enact or even envision alternative forms of belonging and becoming in the city beyond labels like junkie. Senses of being in and out of place were incorporated into the body, fueling symbolic violence and risky regimes of living (Collier and Lakoff 2005)—such as the addict in self-destructive mode who will inevitably hit rock bottom (Bourgois and Schonberg 2009; Vitellone 2004).[7]

Rayna died from an overdose in 2011.

Janet, however, was able to get out. After learning in detox in 2010 that she had hep C, she decided that her best move was to "get the hell out of downtown." Shortly after leaving detox, she took off to Port Coquitlam to meet up with a friend who was squeegeeing (washing car windows at stop lights) there; she didn't spend significant periods of time in downtown Vancouver again for nine years. This geographic transition was accompanied by transitions in both substance use and income generation. In Port Coquitlam, Janet used meth to get off crack and away from sex work (Fast et al. 2014). High on meth, she told me that she roamed the suburbs day and night, meeting new people who were engaged in binning, coppering (stripping copper wiring from empty houses), and other forms of theft, but also landscaping, house painting, and construction work. There, she nurtured new dreams of place. For example, in 2014 she was camping on the edge of a construction site in Port Coquitlam, doing some under the table work on the site. Sitting in a McDonald's restaurant close to where she was sleeping and working, Janet explained that she was choosing to camp outside while she waited for her then-boyfriend of several years, Johnny, to be released from jail. Prior to his incarceration, the two had started a landscaping and house painting business made possible by the truck that Johnny owned.

"I like to have my freedom," she began. "And besides, those places downtown"— she was referring to supportive housing facilities, where a number of those I knew were then living—"don't give you the push you need, to make something of yourself—of your life."

She continued forcefully, "If I'm going to have a place in Vancouver, I'm just gonna see if I can *buy* a house, which is what we're planning on doing when the boyfriend gets out of jail. My boyfriend's got construction work in Fort McMurray for us when he gets out.[8] Has a place lined up for us to live and everything. Anywhere between fifteen hundred and two grand, I'll be making [a week]— him for sure two grand—and we'll probably be staying up there for a good couple of months. So that when we come back, we'll have twenty thousand easy, to put into our business and toward buying a house. And we're actually planning on tying the knot, too," she gushed happily.

Janet told me she had been using more meth than usual to deal with the stress of Johnny being in jail and being on her own. But toward the end of our conversation, she explained, "When I find out when he is *actually* getting out of jail, that week before, I'll detox myself, 'cause I know he's been staying clean in there. And that way, we can just take off for, like, Fort McMurray and not, like, have to worry about anything. Even though he's already talking about using when he gets out, though," Janet frowned. "But maybe we'll just pick up a little bit and take it with us. And then that will be it, right? Because I *do* want to have a kid with him and I know drugs is the main issue for the infertility thing, so. We were talking about that. We were talking about it," she reassured me, and perhaps herself as well.

TRAJECTORIES

Senses of place in the city exerted powerful and transformative effects on young people's trajectories, including their addictions (Raikhel and Garriott 2013b).[9] It was the terrain through which dominant representations of class, race, and pathology organized consent by becoming embodied (Mehta and Bondi 1999). A sense of belonging on the streets and within the poverty management and public health infrastructures of the downtown core shaped ways of being at the most intimate level, including substance use practices (Bourgois and Schonberg 2009). In some moments, young people concluded that their current circumstances were just the way things were—and had always been—for people like them in places like downtown Vancouver, foreclosing other dreams of place. They would always find themselves getting lost and going nowhere in places like hometowns, reserves, hospitals, jails, SROs, supportive housing buildings, and the streets. These moments, when "the future was, strictly speaking, futureless" (Meyers 2013, 114), often coincided with drug binges, relapses and overdoses, the contraction of blood-borne infections, and mental breakdowns.[10]

However, their trajectories in and beyond the city did not simply reflect experience as it had been constituted for them by larger processes of political economy and power. In many moments, their desires for things to be otherwise could crack through apparently rigid social formations and fields and open up new senses of place and self (Biehl and Locke 2017a). Young people were constantly escaping determinants and definitions and enacting various lines of flight into uncertain futures (Deleuze 1997, 2006). Experimentality, improvisation, escape, and flight were perhaps engendered by an almost carnivalesque atmosphere in Vancouver's inner city, where liminality was shaped by dramatic spectacles such as the 2010 Olympics, but also by the monthly cycles of excess and want created by Welfare Wednesdays. They were shaped by an acceleration of wealth accumulation and gentrification accompanied by the continual expansion and contraction of the poverty management and public infrastructures in response to successive waves of emergency. Liminality generated underlying affective currents of unease and danger, but also continually opened up new spaces from which to dream. Senses of place and the trajectories they set in motion could be as multiple and shifting as the city itself.

CARLY AND CONNOR, FAMILY, 2009

Carly had taken off from the field office rather abruptly, after asking me if I could hold onto her purse for her. She had said she would be right back. As the hours passed, I had wondered if I should call the police. Was Carly missing? Was she in trouble? But then, seventy-two hours later, she called me from a friend's phone at nine in the morning and asked if we could meet down at the Lighthouse. And could I please bring her purse?

There weren't many people around as I walked down the alleyway toward the entrance of the shelter. As I approached the heavy metal door, I could hear faint conversation and the occasional cough coming from an adjacent outdoor smoking area that was largely concealed by high chain link fencing and blue plastic tarps. It was around eleven thirty in the morning. I could see that many shelter residents were still underneath blankets pulled up tight over their heads in order to block out the overhead fluorescent lights, sleeping. Others were up and about, doing laundry and talking to each other about their plans for the day. Some attempted to keep their voices down. Others, including Carly and her boyfriend Connor, did not. As I approached, I could see that they were extremely worked up, practically shouting back and forth at each other as they frantically attempted to organize their things on a table half covered with their laundry.

"Can you get my outfit ready?!" Carly asked Connor. "And can you find the *exact* address of the MCFD [Ministry of Children and Family Development] office up on Kingsway [Street]?!"

"Where is my f-cking phone charger?!" Connor replied.

I offered to help look up the address and transit timetables on my phone.

"Today we find out if we get our daughter back," Carly told me, grabbing her purse out of my hands. She burst into tears. "It's now or never."

When I met Carly and Connor in 2008 they had just begun their attempt to regain custody of their one-year-old daughter. Over the following five years, I watched as they had, and lost custody of, another child and continued to navigate the home- and self-making projects mandated by child protective services. The lists of goals that Carly obsessively wrote and rewrote in her journal during this period looked something like this:

Go to residential treatment.
Find a place to live.
Get the money for the first month's rent plus a damage deposit.
Find employment to pay for all of the things that you need to fill a home with.
Go to food banks and drop-in programs to get what you can't afford.
Fill in all of the paperwork for various kinds of social assistance.
Phone the welfare office to get the monthly $20 crisis grant.
Attend daily Twelve Step meetings and do daily step work.
Attend each and every scheduled meeting with social workers, probation officers, doctors, drug and alcohol counselors, and housing agencies.
Attend each and every scheduled supervised visit with your kids.
Do not miss or arrive late to even one of these meetings.
Do not lose your cool in these meetings. Ever.

Between 2009 and 2013, I often accompanied Carly and Connor as they traversed an elaborate geography of meetings, appointments, and chores across Greater Vancouver. In a single day we might take the bus from a shelter in the Downtown South to a drop-in center for young mothers in the Downtown Eastside so that Carly could see her doctor and pick up a donated food bag. Then we would travel by SkyTrain and bus to a suburb so that she and Connor could look at a potential apartment, or to Kingsway Street for an appointment with their social worker, or to Coquitlam for a visit with their kids, being cared for by the same foster family. After that we would travel back downtown so that Carly, at least, could attend a Twelve Step meeting—Connor was much more ambivalent about getting off the crack they both used—before heading back to a shelter. Whenever possible, Carly used any extra money that she and Connor were able to pull together to stay at a cheap, forty-dollar-a-night bed and breakfast. This seemed to annoy their steady rotation of social workers, who felt that they should stay in free shelters and save money. As a solution, Carly and Connor also occasionally slept in Carly's parents' van when it was parked outside the latter's single-story, bungalow-style house in a suburb of Greater Vancouver. During these stays, Carly and Connor entered the house only to use the bathroom, to avoid Carly's parents' open crack use.

"I don't want to get comfortable in the system," Carly told me whenever the issue of where to stay while they were "pulling their lives together" came up. "It's so easy to get sucked in. And then, like, maybe, um, eventually you never get out?"

Carly's and Connor's home- and self-making projects were endlessly complicated by the everyday emergencies of entrenched poverty, unstable housing and homelessness, addiction, and multiple health crises. Connor was schizophrenic, and his behavior could become highly erratic when he missed his monthly shot of long-acting antipsychotic medication. Carly struggled with periods of dramatic weight gain and was perpetually sick with a bad virus or infection. She told me she had experienced crushing periods of depression for as long as she could remember and was prone to an overwhelming desire to sleep for many, many hours a day. The sedating effects of the high dose of methadone that she was on only exasperated this urge, and she struggled to "keep herself going" day after day.

Carly and Connor said that they used crack to wake up from the sedating effects of their medications and for release from various demands and devastating losses. The pressures they were facing could seem contradictory, creating a painful sense of frustration and confusion. On the one hand, they were told by social workers to get out of the system: to find market rental housing and get jobs. On the other, they were told to stay in it: to use free shelters and maintain their eligibility for things like subsidized bus passes. They were told to create a home for their kids, which neither of them could easily imagine doing without the other, but also that they would need to separate to attend residential treatment programs as a condition for regaining custody. Eventually, Carly was told that she would need to separate from Connor completely if she wanted a chance to regain custody independently during her extended periods of sobriety.

Many times when I met up with them Carly admitted tearfully that she had relapsed, and Connor admitted somewhat more coldly that he had never really stopped using. "Sometimes we just can't hold it together anymore," Carly often reflected. "You break down. And then, it's just like, why bother anymore? Everything just seems to be against us. So, you just decide to keep going [with drugs], because really, where else are you going in life?"

And yet, across multiple relapses, again and again Carly vowed to get herself going and do everything she needed to do to get her kids back. She never completely gave up on her dream of creating a family with Connor and their kids, even if her sense of momentum waxed and waned. Tragically, it seemed that Connor's central place in this dream was what prevented the other aspects of it from being realized.

Connor talked to me often about how much he had loved being a dad and husband (although the couple was not legally married) during the relatively brief times when he and Carly had custody of their children. He reflected that he had frequently been the children's primary caregiver when Carly struggled with periods of depression and excessive somnolence. However, over the years Connor was unwilling to cease his crack use to regain custody. He was unapologetic about his continued drug use, much as Carly was unapologetic about her continued relationship with Connor, even as their social workers issued stern warnings about both.

"I'm still using because I don't have my kids, right?" Connor explained to me in late 2013. By this time, he was living in his own room in a supportive housing building to fulfil a social worker's stipulation that he and Carly live separately. "And I figure I may as well use until I get my kids back and then when I *do* get my kids back I'll stop—like, I can do that, right?"

He paused. "I just want my family back. But like, right now? I have nothing to fill my time with. Like, I don't have kids to feed and bathe and clothe right now. The ministry has gotten their way and broken me and Carly apart [in the sense of living in two separate places]. So, every single day right now, it's a matter of going, okay, what do I do now? It's either come home from work and go to sleep at six o'clock at night and then wake up for work and then come home and then go to sleep again, or it's come home from work and enjoy a high for three or four hours and then go to sleep and then go to work. Right? I have no TV in my room. No cable. All I can do is sit there and stare at the walls. Unless I have the drugs," he added.

GEOGRAPHIES

Young people refused to confine their dreams of place to downtown Vancouver. Most also refused to physically stay put in these neighborhoods, moving back and forth—sometimes several times a day—between the downtown core and other areas of the city. And so while this project may have started in downtown Vancouver, it quickly expanded. A significant amount of my time with them was spent on the move, traveling via public buses and the SkyTrain between various nodes of social, economic, and institutional activity. These included the bustling transportation hub at Broadway and Commercial Street in East Vancouver; the crack shacks, flop houses, informal recovery houses, and camps scattered throughout the suburbs of Surrey, Port Coquitlam, New Westminster, and Burnaby; shoplifting hot spots like Metrotown Mall and Lougheed Town Centre; and the Kingsway sex work stroll.[11] Young people's movements through the city were also shaped by elaborate geographies of Twelve Step meetings and endless appointments with social workers, housing workers, welfare workers, probation officers, drug and alcohol counselors, and doctors. Tracing their movements through the city and across intimate and institutional domains allowed me to attend not only to their everyday experiences but also to the material out of which those experiences were made, which included various technologies of administration and the self (Foucault 1997a).

PATTY AND JOE, HOME, 2012

"One day, I'd like to live in one of those nice condos down by the beach," Patty said in 2012. "In English Bay. Yeah. I love it there."

After a moment, Patty continued thoughtfully, "Just to be able to feel like we're not in the system anymore. Me and Joe, living in a regular building with regular residents. And, I don't know, maybe then I'd want to go back to school—be able to focus on school, and everything? Finish my high school and get my diploma, and then pick a career from there." She and her boyfriend, Joe, smiled at each other, seeming to take comfort in repeating to me—and to themselves—the plan that they had been living on the edge of for so many years.

Joe was characteristically agreeable. "Yeah, that's where I would say I'd want to live, too," he chimed in. "In the West End. I like the ocean. And I like being able to see the mountains."

"We always stick together," Patty laughed. "We're lucky in that way."

When I first met Patty and Joe in 2008 they were living in a small camp underneath the bridge that links the Downtown South and Kitsilano neighborhoods of Vancouver. Their camp was a peaceful place, surrounded by dense foliage, almost directly on the beach: you could hear the sounds of the ocean from their small, battered tent. No one ever seemed to bother them there. Each day, Patty and Joe would travel from this camp into the Downtown South to access various services and drop-in programs for street youth. In 2008 Patty was red zoned (legally barred) from virtually all of downtown Vancouver and was in and out of city jail frequently.[12] At that time she and Joe were making money however they could: panhandling, shoplifting, doing robberies, flipping traded and stolen merch, engaging in street-level drug dealing and sex work, and participating in a street youth job program that mostly involved picking up garbage off the down-town sidewalks.[13] Her red zones didn't stop Patty from going to the Downtown South every day. "I need these [service] places," she stated firmly.

In 2008 Patty and Joe were avoiding the Downtown Eastside neighborhood, but not because of Patty's red zones. When I first met Patty she had just returned to Vancouver again after a trip back home to Edmonton. Patty had been living and sleeping outside in Edmonton, too, much as she had done throughout her adolescence as she cycled between group homes and juvenile detention facilities in that Canadian city. But this recent stay in Edmonton—even if she was on the streets there—had allowed her to take a break from the "drama" of intensive drug use and debts, which had turned increasingly violent in Vancouver prior to her departure. Like so many others, Patty understood the Downtown Eastside to be the epicenter of this drama and its associated violence.

Over the years I knew her Patty, perhaps more than any other young person I knew, questioned whether she truly belonged in Vancouver. On the one hand, she shared the same dreams of place as many others, and I watched as she worked tirelessly to make a home for herself and Joe in the city. On the other hand, Patty thought constantly about leaving Vancouver and wanted Joe to do the same. Patty and Joe both maintained regular phone contact with family members in other provinces, and Patty told me often that her real dream was to travel or even move permanently back home so that she could more fully reconnect with her family and make big changes in her life. Joe was much more ambivalent about returning to his hometown in the province of Saskatchewan. And Patty was ambivalent about leaving Joe without an exit plan of his own.

As time passed Patty became increasingly anxious about realizing this dream. "I don't want to wake up one day and realize it's too late," she told me in 2013. She explained that returning home would be a means of slowing down her drug use. This project would become all the more urgent with the arrival of illicitly manu-factured fentanyl and related analogues in the local drug supply sometime in 2011 and the steady escalation of an unprecedented overdose crisis in the years fol-lowing. By the time an official overdose public health emergency was declared by the Government of BC in 2016, Patty, like so many others, was living on the edge of death.

However, Patty often seemed to be in a state of suspension between finally returning home and feeling like she could not leave Vancouver and Joe just yet. I came to think that this state of suspension was perhaps shaped by the compli-cated tides of her desires for the future and painful memories of the past. Patty longed to develop closer relationships with her grandparents and parents, but her movements between Vancouver and Edmonton were also layered with memories of her daughter, Shayley, who had been removed from her custody when Patty was seventeen and Shayley was ten months old. It was when she lost custody of Shayley that Patty fled to Vancouver for the first time, using the child benefit money that she had been owed by the government. Patty told me once that she probably could have gotten Shayley back if she had been able to do "every little thing the social workers were asking for—all of the paperwork, and meetings, and appointments"—but in the end she "just didn't make it."

Patty very rarely mentioned Shayley to me, and she never came out and said that painful memories of her daughter were a part of what had prevented her from returning home. But in 2016 Patty finally took a trip back to Edmonton. She went seemingly on a whim when her grandparents sent her the money (and then sent her the money again) for a bus ticket. Patty had wanted Joe to go to detox while she was away, so that he could "clean up" a bit. He had ultimately refused, yet this time Patty had managed to tear herself away from the fragile world they shared.

During our first meeting after Patty had arrived back in Vancouver from her trip home in 2016, I came to more deeply appreciate how memories of Shayley had perhaps shaped Patty's dreams and fears of returning to Edmonton. Patty spoke to me for the first time at length about Shayley and what kind of mom she had been during those first ten months. While she had been staying in the basement of her grandparents' house, Patty found an old Ziploc bag containing a single baby photo of Shayley and their matching hospital bracelets from when she was born. Sitting together in the field office, Patty carefully placed the photograph and bracelets on the table in front of us. She picked up each object again and again and encouraged me to do the same, telling me how happy she was to have these objects in her possession again after all these years. Her relief—the sense that some sort of huge weight had been lifted—was palpable.

"Going home, was, like, actually kind of scary in a way?" Patty admitted toward the end of our conversation. Her tone was uncertain. She took a long, deep breath. "But I'm actually feeling, like, much more at peace with everything now." She fingered the worn edges of the baby photo. "I remembered a lot when I was home. And, like, not just the bad stuff. I remembered that when I was pregnant with Shayley, and even, like, after I had her and stuff, I was doing really good. It was a really good time in my life. Me and my boyfriend lived on our own [in Edmonton]. We had our own apartment and everything. And I was going to, um, Sprott-Shaw Community College? I did this program where they pay you if you have good attendance. I had a lot of money, actually!" She laughed. "I was, like, two and a half years clean. Bought, like, tons of baby stuff. And Shayley still has it all, I bet," Patty imagined. She smiled widely and wrapped her arms tightly around herself, as if in an embrace.

PART 2 SOMETHING

PATTY, COAST SALISH TERRITORIES, 2009

"Down here—all this?" Patty gestured around the Lighthouse shelter, which was humming with the kind of energy that lurched constantly between ecstatic and menacing. "This is *something* I have, right? At least it's *something*. Something that fills my time, basically."

Across the unceded and occupied Coast Salish Territories of the Sḵwx̱wú7mesh, səlilwətaʔɬ, and xʷməθkʷəy̓əm First Nations, young bodies pulsed with the intensities of memories, dreams, and desires and meth, crack, and heroin.

VITAL EXPERIMENTATION

Substance use in the context of entrenched poverty and homelessness continues to be primarily framed in terms of risk and harm. It is also viewed as a means of coping and self-medication for physical, psychological, emotional, economic, and historical injuries and intergenerational trauma. Yet this is not the whole story. Young people's substance use could equally be a process of vital experimentation (Deleuze 2007) that might open up new social, economic, spatial, and affective possibilities, even as it could turn dangerous or deadly and powerfully constrain life chances (Pine 2019; Raikhel and Garriott 2013b).[1]

Drug use as a form of vital experimentation was inseparable from the embodied, affective senses of place they experienced across time. Painful experiences of boredom and stagnation in the places of their childhoods and in the City of Vancouver were mediated by the intensive consumption of drugs and alcohol, which often enmeshed them in new affective intensities that included a powerful sense of forward momentum or being at the center of *something* rife with potential for movement of some kind. Addiction embroiled those I followed in frenetic cycles of using drugs, needing more drugs, and working to track down money, drugs, and the people who had both, while simultaneously avoiding police, red zones, and those to whom they owed money. These cycles could encompass a few square blocks in the downtown core or expansive urban geographies across various suburbs of Greater Vancouver. Even as substance use exacerbated marginalization, addiction nevertheless propelled young people forward each day in the sense that there was always another all-consuming mission (to track down drugs, the money for drugs, or the people who had both), another interpersonal drama (often connected to tracking down people, money, and drugs), and another high on the horizon. Substances held them together, tore them apart, and brought them back together. They kept them moving through the city, on foot and via public transit.

And then there were the affective intensities of substances themselves.

"Crack is a more, more, more, more, more drug."
"Crack is a drug that doesn't end."
"You just keep going and going and going and using it and using it and using it."
"Meth gets you up and motivates you to be productive."
"Meth makes you feel like you can do anything."[2]
"Meth kills your depression."
"Meth makes you feel like a normal person."
"It lasts ages and ages and ages."
"Alcohol balances the up, up, up feeling of the meth."
"Alcohol calms you down."
"Heroin is like a blanket that wraps around you."
"Doing heroin makes you feel like you are melting into nothingness."
"Heroin lets you finally sleep."
"And then you're doing the same thing over and over and over and over again to
     get more and more and more and more."
"Drugs can make every other part of life feel boring."

SHAE, LULA, AND JEFF, LIGHTHOUSE SHELTER, 2009

Shae met me at the entrance to the Lighthouse shelter. It was a warm evening in the spring of 2009, the late afternoon sunlight casting a golden hue on every surface it touched. Shae had dropped into the field office earlier that day as they so often did and said they had loads to tell me. Would I like to drop by the Lighthouse after work? As I walked down the hill from the field office toward the shelter, it seemed like the entire city was outside enjoying what felt like the first real day of summer. When I turned down the alleyway that led to the shelter entrance, I saw that the residents of the Lighthouse were no exception. The alley was buzzing with activity.

Funded by the province, the City of Vancouver, and a private foundation and operated by a local social housing agency, the Lighthouse was located in a derelict, single-story building directly underneath the Granville Street Bridge. It was perpetually in shadow, but from the back alley it had a much grander feel. For a time in 2008 and 2009, this alley was one of the most notorious drug-dealing spots in the Downtown South. Through the heavy metal door that was the shelter's only entrance and exit, young people slammed in and out of the building with teenage intensity. Loud conversations and arguments could be heard on both sides of the door, as they bought and sold drugs, struck up drug-dealing partnerships and romantic relationships, and resolved debts and other kinds of drama. In a yard that ran down the length of the building, tarps were strung up across high chain link fencing, sectioning off a prized smoking area that was, everyone boasted at the time, "off limits to cops." Inside the shelter, mattresses and bedding were lined up in neat rows, with personal belongings stored in large plastic tubs. Those who had been at the Lighthouse the longest had secured coveted spots along the edges of the room, where they decorated the walls adjacent to their mattresses with pages torn out of coloring books, drawings, photographs, and other keepsakes. In the evenings, couples pushed their mattresses together.

As I approached the entrance to the shelter that evening, I saw that Lula was standing with Shae, their heads bent together in urgent, whispered conversation. Jeff was nowhere to be seen, but a short distance away Patty and Joe were standing with Laurie and Aaron and two other young men I didn't know, talking and laughing loudly together. Aaron and one of the men started play fighting, pulling each other to the ground. A small axe with a plastic cover over the blade fell out of one of their jackets. Aaron picked it up and brandished it menacingly. Patty and Laurie rolled their eyes and obsessively adjusted each other's hair and outfits. They kept looking up toward the top of the alleyway, clearly waiting for someone.

"I was thinking—today, like, the weather is *exactly* what it was like when I first came here," Shae said, as they led me inside the shelter. "It was sunny and perfect *every single day* like this, for my entire first summer here." Shae moved around the large open room at a brisk, almost feverish pace, gathering up a few belongings and seeming to check and recheck that other things were where they had left them.

I met Shae a year earlier, shortly after they fled to Vancouver following a period of significant family and mental health crisis and involuntary institutionalization in a psychiatric facility in the adjacent province of Alberta. Upon arriving in the city, they quickly integrated themselves into what young people often referred to as the "scene" in downtown Vancouver. Within a matter of weeks in the early summer of 2008, Shae seemed to know everyone and everyone knew them. Many of these individuals quickly became Shae's chosen family. They referred to Lula and Janet as their sisters and Patty as their daughter.

We made our way down to the beach, located just a few blocks from the shelter, so that we could talk in private. Sitting with our backs against a large sun-warmed log and watching the gradually darkening ocean wash up against the shore, Shae reminisced about their "perfect first year in the city."

"All last summer, we just chilled and drank and smoked weed down at English Bay [beach in the West End]. It was—like—magical, almost? And *then*—" Shae became increasingly animated "—on Christmas Day of last year, right? It snowed in just the most *perfect* way. When it, like, rarely snows here, right? It was, like, a sign! Of, like, what this year *is* in my life, right?"

During the previous year, Shae had become increasingly addicted to meth, a substance that they said seemed to make everything in their life "work better." "I have struggled with depression and ADHD *all my life*, okay," Shae said that evening. "But meth has made me be more social, gotten me out of my shell—you know what I mean? When I started using it, it was like, suddenly I wanted to *do* things, wanted to *see* people and be with people, every single day. I'm so much happier than I used to be. And I'm having *way* more fun than I ever have in my entire—whole—life, right?"

After arriving in the city in late spring 2008, Shae spent months sleeping outside and couch surfing until the Lighthouse opened that winter. The opening of the shelter threw many young people together in a new way. While this was not the case for everyone, for Shae and some others the Lighthouse allowed them to create a fragile home and new, complicated families with one another, even in the midst of entrenched poverty, homelessness, and perpetual chaos.

"At the Lighthouse, I have all of my friends and I have my *family* around me, right?" Shae began listing off various relations: "I have my sister Lula. I have my sister Janet. And actually, I'm, like, the mama bear of the group, right? I take care of *everyone*. Patty is my *actual* daughter, because we knew each other from the streets in Edmonton, even before all of this. And I *love* being that, right? The one who takes care of everyone. Even when things get *f-cking crazy*. And they get *crazy*," Shae laughed. "It is honestly nonstop drama with all of these people, right? It's, like, my *full-time job* sorting through all of the problems that happen. I'm not even *joking*." Shae turned to look at me suddenly. "Which brings me to, like—have you *heard* what is happening today with Lula and Jeff? *Oh my god.*"

Lula was threatening to have Jeff sprayed with bear repellent (a common form of violence during the earlier years of my fieldwork) by someone she was insisting he owed money to, even though it was Lula who had borrowed the fifty bucks. When she borrowed the money, she told the person lending it (who was also in the scene) that her boyfriend Jeff owed her that exact amount and that he could collect what he was owed directly from Jeff. Jeff did not agree that he owed Lula that amount of money, nor did he have the money to settle the loan. So now Jeff was potentially going to get "bear sprayed" because he could not pay off the debt.

Lula borrowed the fifty dollars from this individual to buy crack, which was Lula and Jeff's drug of choice when I first met them in 2009. However, Lula also set up this deal with the lender to punish Jeff, with whom she was furious for flailing off from the Lighthouse for hours, during which time she suspected that he had used crack without her. She also suspected, again, that he was cheating on her. Lula wanted and needed Jeff to stay with her, constantly. She wanted and needed him to take care of her, all the time. Jeff, on the other hand, often said that he needed to take breaks from Lula to stay sane.

The Lighthouse was an integral part of Lula and Jeff's love story, although compared to many others I followed, the two were there for only a short period before it was shut down. They met each other walking along Granville Street in early 2009 and fell instantly in love. They stayed together at the shelter for a few short months. During their first month there, Lula spent half of her time in jail on a shoplifting charge. While in jail she couldn't stop thinking about Jeff, and the rest, as Lula put it, was history.

Lula and Jeff seemed to love each other deeply and were together on and off for the entire duration of this project. Like so many others, their union was at the very center of their lives. Over the years, Lula declared and redeclared their engagement and unofficial marriage on Facebook as well as Jeff's various transgressions and their many breakups. They fought constantly and brutally. They screamed at and frequently became violent toward one another, and on too many occasions to count the cops were called to break them apart. Both Jeff and Lula—but mostly Jeff—had been arrested during these altercations. On more than one occasion Jeff likened his suffering and capacity for forgiveness, in the context of his relationship with Lula, to that of Jesus. But he was highly ambivalent about ending things. Instead, he frequently emphasized to me with a tone of pride that at least he was enduring *something*.

About a week after I went down to the beach with Shae I ran into Jeff on Granville Street at one of his usual panhandling spots. He told me that while he had ultimately not gotten bear sprayed over the fifty-dollar debt, he had been arrested and spent a night in city jail after he and Lula had "gone crazy" at each other at the Lighthouse, screaming, fighting, and throwing things. By the time I saw him panhandling, however, they had already made up with Shae's help as mediator.

Jeff reflected, "The police have said that if I stay with Lula, I'm gonna go back to jail over and over again. And that I'm just *asking for it*. But, like, when I do break up with her, or we, like, have time apart? I feel like I have, like, no-no-no—purpose? Or something. I seem to be having a hard time with driving myself forward, if I'm, like, not with her."

Later that week at the Lighthouse, Lula likewise said to me, "I don't know what to *do with myself* if I'm not with Jeff, and, like, caught up in all of this. Honestly, life is just so boring that way. And then I get into even more trouble."

Over the years I watched as the drama between Lula and Jeff propelled them forward day after day. They loved each other. They hated each other. One of them was in jail because of an altercation between them. One of them had taken off somewhere because of an altercation between them. Jeff had a new girlfriend whom Lula hated. Lula had a new fiancé whom Jeff hated. Jeff had to take care of Lula no matter what. Lula couldn't live without Jeff. After the Lighthouse shelter was closed in summer 2009 and they began cycling through various SROs and supportive housing buildings, they were barred from each other's residences over and over again. They would sneak each other in, resulting in frequent altercations with building staff and numerous evictions. These were always devastating, but they heightened the drama between them even further.

The churn of drama between Lula and Jeff was fueled by the stimulating effects of their use of crack and later meth, to which they both transitioned by 2012. Episodes of what young people often summarized as "going crazy" and "acting psycho" were also fueled by mental health challenges, including substance-use-induced paranoia and hallucinations. Jeff told me he had ADHD and depression. Lula said she had been diagnosed with schizoaffective and anxiety disorders and depression. But to reduce the drama of substance use and romantic relationships to young people's mental health and addictions perhaps misses its vital, affective dimensions. This drama was *something* in which those I followed were deeply immersed. It gave them a powerful sense of forward momentum and expanded to fill their time.

Over the first several years of our acquaintance, whenever we spent time together, Lula and Jeff were always charged up. Like Shae, I often found myself refereeing screaming matches. And then in 2015 Jeff dramatically reduced his meth use and began using heroin/fentanyl intensively.[3] He also started to go on and off methadone. His demeanor was completely transformed by this transition. At least when the three of us were together, his loud, oftentimes aggressive way of speaking to Lula (and sometimes to me as well) was replaced by soft-spokenness. He moved more slowly, with an air of general contentedness, even when Lula railed at him. Jeff's transformation seemed to dissipate some of the drama between them. He was no longer in and out of jail on charges related to his fights with Lula, at least. And yet a new element of discord had been introduced into their relationship. Lula, who continued to use meth intensively and would often stay awake for days at a time, disliked how Jeff seemed to be increasingly sinking into sedation and sleep when he was not out hustling for money and drugs.

"I miss the old Jeff," Lula admitted to me at the end of 2015. "He never wants to *do* anything anymore, except when he's on the grind [trying to make money]. Like, that's the only thing that gets him going anymore. He doesn't even *want to have sex*."

MOMENTUM

The rhythms, routines, and affective intensities of addiction—and perhaps in particular addictions to meth and crack—could give young people a powerful sense of forward momentum. Their embroilment in what they frequently referred to as the drama of romantic relationships and friendships, drug dealing, debts, and crime can also be understood in relation to a sense of momentum or being at the center of something rife with potential (Karandinos et al. 2014).[4]

We can draw on materialist arguments to explain how and why young people become embroiled in oftentimes volatile relationships and forms of income generation. In the context of romantic relationships and friendships on the streets, the reciprocal sharing of material resources and emotional and physical support incurs mutual debts that equip individuals to better navigate the everyday emergencies of entrenched poverty, unstable housing, homelessness, and addiction (Bourgois and Schonberg 2009). Similarly, embroilment in drug dealing, debts, and crime is shaped by the imperatives of addiction and day-to-day survival in the context of extreme poverty. Involvement in these often also powerfully intersects with more expansive desires. These include the "search for respect" (Bourgois 1996) and recognition (Henry 2015, 2019) in postindustrial and settler-colonial cities, as well as the "renegade dreams" that transform various kinds of urban physical, social, and economic injury into aspirations for different kinds of futures (Ralph 2014).

However, these framings fail to capture how such endeavors also generate particular affective intensities that seemed to be at the heart of what it meant to live a good—or at least worthwhile—life among those I followed (Robbins 2013). Money and status were certainly important to young people (see also Henry 2015, 2019), but they were fleeting at best. Most rose to glory in the low-level drug-dealing "game" and other criminal enterprises, only to descend again into destitution and debt. Reputations were built and annihilated with the same speed. These cycles of feast and famine did not necessarily undermine a sense of momentum or being at the center of something, however. For many, they amplified it. Those I knew often remarked that they were as addicted to the "rush" of dealing and crime—including those moments when the game was up and they had to start back from square one—as they were to the substances that they put into their bodies. They also talked about being addicted to the drama of their romantic relationships, even as this was also a source of suffering in their lives. They told me that without this rush, without this drama they would have nothing to fill their lives with. A powerful sense of possibility was generated by the constant need to problem solve and make things work against all odds. Along with intensive forms of substance use, this was the *something* in which they were embroiled.

LAURIE AND AARON, TRAFALGAR HOTEL, 2010

I almost didn't recognize Laurie as she greeted me at the front door of the Trafalgar Hotel at the beginning of March 2010. She had cut her hair into a short mohawk and dyed the tips bright orange. "You can pay $500 for a haircut like this in Hollywood," she said with a sly smile. "But I paid $139 for this *and* my eyebrows. Aaron gave me the money." Laurie loved hair and fashion and talked occasionally about going to hairdressing or design school. That day she was wearing a tight black tank top and loose pink terry cloth sweat pants. One of her bright red bra straps was hung down purposively around her tiny bicep. Laurie was extraordinarily petite, but she knew how to take up a lot of space. When she walked down the hallways of the Trafalgar or the streets of the downtown core, people tended to move out of her way. Her boyfriend, Aaron, was exactly the same: short and small boned but with a large, intimidating presence.

Laurie and Aaron had already been together for a year when I met them in 2008, and they would stay together until 2016. They first encountered each other while using the computers in downtown Vancouver's large public library and fell quickly in love. They stayed together at the Lighthouse shelter, and after it was closed down were moved into Trafalgar Hotel, a government-owned but yet-to-be-renovated SRO located only a few blocks away. The third-floor room that Laurie unofficially shared with Aaron in the Trafalgar was miniscule, filthy, and crammed with stuff. That day in March I had to push a chair against the door to make a place for myself to sit, while Laurie waded through piles of clothes, shoes, coloring books, markers, toiletries, makeup, junk food wrappers, and empty drink bottles to join Aaron on a double mattress that took up almost half the room. As small as these rooms were, I had frequently seen five or six individuals packed into them for extended periods.

Hanging on Laurie's wall beside her mattress was a 2010 calendar that meticulously documented her day-to-day substance use. Each time I visited her over the course of that year I asked if I could look at it with her. I also asked to see the calendars that she had kept for 2008 and 2009, which were carefully stored in a large blue Rubbermaid tub that had come with her to the Trafalgar from the Lighthouse. Laurie's calendars told a story about her substance use across time as well as her relationship with Aaron (see also Meyers 2013). When I met the couple in 2008 they were both drinking and using crack intensively. They also used meth occasionally. Then, in 2009, Aaron slowly replaced his crack use with more intensive meth use (Fast et al. 2014), while Laurie continued to use crack—much to Aaron's displeasure. When Laurie and Aaron were not getting along, Laurie would take off from the Downtown South to the Downtown Eastside to binge on crack and alcohol for a few days. She often didn't remember what happened and would fill out her calendar with the words "crack" and "booze" and the descriptor "BLACKOUT!" as best as she could after the fact.

On at least two of these occasions Laurie had ended up in hospital: once as a result of an overdose and once from a beating she had received. During these hospitalizations the doctors warned her that she had significant liver damage and needed to stop drinking, but it was the news of Aaron's biological mom's death from alcoholism in late 2009 that finally convinced both Laurie and Aaron to quit drinking. The two of them detoxed themselves off alcohol while living at the Trafalgar. The word "DETOX" was written in capital letters across fourteen days of the calendar page for December 2009. Going over this page with me, Laurie said that both she and Aaron had horrible tremors during their self-detox. Laurie even "saw lights" a couple of times during the process, leading me to wonder whether she had a seizure. Nevertheless, they were now thrilled that they had been able to successfully "do it on their own" rather than check themselves into a medical detox, and more than two months later neither of them seemed to be drinking. "That's *f-cking strong*," Laurie boasted with her usual bravado. "We didn't need anybody's help, you know? Me and Aaron did it together because we are both *soldiers*, you know what I mean?"

Since she stopped drinking, Laurie's calendar revealed that she had begun using meth more intensively. It also showed that, by the end of January 2010, she had completely stopped using crack. Laurie seemed very happy with this transition, which Aaron had been urging her toward for almost a year. "With jib [a slang term for meth], you *function*," she said. "All my friends, my family, my crew—they're all so, like, proud of me for stopping the drinking *and* the crack, right? On jib I'm, like, able to go and run around every day and do what I need to do and *think straight*—now. It's so awesome. And my relationship is *way* stronger now, too."

"Do you agree with that, Aaron?" I asked. He had thus far remained silent during our conversation, typing rapidly on a battered phone that he had not had the last time I saw him and Laurie. Among most of those I knew, phones like this came and went frequently.

"Yeah," he said distractedly, not looking at me. "I'm happy that we stopped drinking, because I lost my mom to that, right? Even though I didn't really know my mom. And, like, I'm happy that Laurie is off the crack, too, right? Because I didn't like who she was on it, at all. We were, like, fighting all the time, right? I gotta go, though," he said suddenly, grabbing an oversized jacket and getting up from the mattress. I moved my chair aside so that he could squeeze through the door. He gave Laurie a pointed look and said, "I gotta go downstairs. To deal with some business."

"He's gotta go to work now," Laurie said triumphantly after Aaron had left. "For the boss."

During his time at the Lighthouse and the Trafalgar, and then in the various SROs and supportive housing buildings that he cycled through from there, I observed that Aaron was a key player in the low-level drug-dealing game that was constantly unfolding. As he liked to put it, he moved in and took over, over and over again. Alternatively, whenever Laurie tried her hand at dealing, she ended up "doing her own product" and racking up debts that Aaron then had to pay off. While Laurie and Aaron were not made members of a well-established Indigenous street gang originating in eastern Canada, they had biological family members residing in Vancouver who were.[5] This meant that they usually had a "hookup" to moderate quantities of drugs to sell. Alongside low-level dealing, for almost two years while he was living at the Lighthouse shelter and Trafalgar Hotel Aaron also picked up under-the-table bar work at a local strip club. I got the sense that he had very low tolerance for being without regular income in addition to his monthly social assistance check. Laurie, by association, seemed to share this intolerance for being broke and on the grind every day of the month except Welfare Wednesday and the few days that followed. She would often list off to me in detail the large and small things that Aaron provided her with because of his financial prowess—the various junk foods on which they both seemed to subsist, money to get her hair and eyebrows done, knockoff designer purses. She also regularly derided those couples not able to provide for each other the way that Aaron was able to provide for her.

Romantic relationships, friendships, and drug-dealing partnerships previously established at the Lighthouse shelter, however volatile, appeared to survive moves to hotels like the Trafalgar and the Mackenzie. This continued to be described as a time when everyone knew everyone and young people "ran things"—from various illegal income-generation schemes inside buildings to doing their own harm reduction and outreach. Intervention by building staff was almost nonexistent, even though both hotels were by this time owned by the state. Drugs were bought, sold, and used openly within buildings. Crime and violence were rampant. Both the Trafalgar and Mackenzie hotels were dirty and bug-infested, with sinks and shared toilets that became clogged and overflowed. This was often described by young people in hindsight as a "crazy" time, as in "crazy dangerous" but also "crazy fun."

"Our door got kicked in last week," Laurie said as I readjusted my chair again so that I was sitting directly in front of it. I had noticed when we came in that the door was basically falling off its hinges. "That's the *third* time it's happened since moving here." She sounded more excited than alarmed. As if on cue, a loud argument erupted in the hallway, and someone began pounding on a different door a short distance down the hallway.

"Someone trying to rob us!" Laurie continued, becoming increasingly loud and animated. "But me and Aaron know *exactly* who did it, and when we catch him, it's *go time*!" She began pacing back and forth on the mattress, the coffee I had brought her teetering precariously in her hand as she almost lost her footing. "Because he doesn't get *who* he just messed with, right? Oh! And Aaron got bear sprayed, right? Did you hear about that?!" I had already heard the story but didn't stop Laurie from launching into it again. I had long ago noticed that the telling and retelling of stories like this was itself a way of generating a sense of momentum and being at the center of something. The overall gist was that Aaron had been taken by surprise and attacked only a few blocks away from the Trafalgar by someone who was insisting that Aaron owed him money. The debt was related to a drug-dealing partnership that the two of them had struck up for a few days, which involved pooling their initial investment of funds and sharing any profits.

Laurie concluded, "The guy who bear sprayed him, right? He was actually just a little guy, too. Like, not much bigger than me and Aaron! And you know what, we actually give him *a lot* of respect, because he has *a lot of heart* for a little guy, right? But my friend has the guy who bear sprayed Aaron on Facebook. We have *already* identified him. So now we just need to figure out where he is hiding. Because he has to take a beating now, right?"

"Do you ever feel scared, living here?" I asked. "Like even right now—there's something going on in the hallway—"

"No," Laurie cut me off. "We *run* things in here. We have our crew. We stick together, right? Make money together. *No one can f-ck with us!*" Laurie yelled, so that anyone within earshot in the hallway could hear her. "And especially not me and Aaron, because of our family connections down here, right?"

"Right," I said uncertainly. I was thinking of how Laurie had been very badly hurt not that long ago while on a crack and alcohol binge in the Downtown Eastside.

Laurie continued, "All of this, right? It's the *hustle*. The *game*. And then there's the drama on top of that, right? *Family* drama!" Laurie laughed. "But, like, we mostly sort it out, right? Just like a family. You hear something, and then go talk about it face to face so that you aren't playing—you know that game telephone? And yeah, like, sometimes someone has to take a beating, right? Everyone knows that's just the way it is. Because they did something they shouldn't. Owed someone money. Hooked up with the wrong person. But, like, even when you, like, take that beating, there's actually *a lot* of pride in that, right? You get respect."

"It sounds like you are liking it here," I said, still uncertain about what questions to ask. "I was kind of worried about how things might change—you know, when the Lighthouse closed down."

"The shelter was *fun!*" Laurie exclaimed. "Getting drunk, walking to Stanley Park! Running around all day and night! Just being together, and just, like, helping each other out, right? But, like, yeah, we love the Trafalgar, too. For the most part. *Sooooooooooo* many good times here, too. There are so many of us together here too, still. And we all, like, click. We're a family. Me and Aaron have made another home here, I think."

Laurie had told me once, not long after we first met, that she was a person with a lot of homes. But both she and Aaron had made it clear to me that they actively worked to block deeply painful memories of their pasts, and therefore I rarely asked them about how they had grown up. However, certain memories did surface in our conversations over the years. They both told me a small amount about experiences of cycling through government group and foster homes throughout their childhoods and the agony of both longing for their birth parents and needing to get away from tumultuous home environments. One time, Laurie told me about her sister, who had moved with her through various government homes until she died at fifteen years of age. She also told me about her first serious boyfriend, who had died as a result of gang-connected violence when they were both sixteen. Laurie said that these losses shaped her alcoholism; she had started drinking more heavily when her sister died, and it was a part of what got her through the subsequent death of her boyfriend. Both Laurie and Aaron spent much of their childhoods and adolescences running away again and again from government homes and the profound losses embedded in these places. They lived everywhere and nowhere, as Aaron once put it. It was on the streets of Vancouver that they finally stopped running and instead began to make a home and family with each other.

Eventually, Aaron returned to the room. He was clearly worked up, and I took that as my cue to leave. As I was turning off my recorder and organizing some money to give to Laurie for her time, the two attempted to have a hushed, quiet conversation in the opposite corner of the tiny room. But Laurie was amped up and kept raising her voice. It was clear that Aaron thought he knew where the guy who had bear sprayed him was hiding, and he and Laurie and a number of others were now going to go and track him down near the Broadway and Commercial intersection in East Vancouver.

"Me and Aaron gotta put on our game faces now!" Laurie exclaimed as I stood up to leave. She began pacing the mattress again while simultaneously touching up her heavy eye makeup.

"What does that mean?" I asked.

"It's a different face, when you're going to go do your thing on the street in front of everybody, right? That's a different face you put on. When it's just me and Aaron—like, someone I can completely trust? I can chill, I can relax, I can slow down a bit." Aaron laughed at this. I got the sense that Laurie rarely slowed down these days.

"But out there?" she continued. "No weakness. No emotions. Just your game face."

"Never a dull moment, right?" Aaron said, chuckling softly. "Just how me and Laurie like it."

MORAL WORLDS

Drug dealing, debts, crime, and romantic relationships generated a powerful sense of momentum and possibility. They also opened up new value systems and logics, anchoring elaborate moral worlds that issued particular kinds of "unavoidable demands" (Zigon 2013, 201) in particular moments.[6] Much of the drama in which young people were immersed was generated by their attempts to elaborate, embody, and defend these moral worlds.

I spent a great deal of my time with them listening to animated and oftentimes fantastical narratives of dealing-, debt-, and crime-related achievements and defeats and endless gossip about what was happening in their own and other people's romantic relationships (and, to a lesser extent, friendships). The conclusions to be drawn from these stories—their undying love for one another, their irredeemable disappointment and anger, the need for swift retribution—were also etched across the walls of their rooms and the various buildings that they passed by and sheltered beneath each day. These modes of storytelling were a way of clarifying understandings of right and wrong and the behaviors that should follow from them.

Stay together with your romantic partner no matter what.
Take care of each other.
Provide for each other.
Binge on drugs together.
Detox together.
Recover together.
Don't separate, no matter what.
Even if that means not going to residential treatment or detox.
Even if that means not getting your kids back from the ministry.[7]

Romantic relationships were one intelligible site of moral reasoning and ethical action. The gang was another (Henry 2019). While most of those I followed were not members of local gangs, they all fiercely embraced particular moral logics of the gang, which they often seemed to glean from popular films as much as from acquaintances, friends, and family members who were gang members.[8] Regular involvement in low-level, loosely gang-connected dealing and other forms of crime and frequent periods of time spent in jail—or being in a romantic relationship with someone who was traversing this trajectory—brought most I knew into close proximity with these logics.

Be a loyal worker.
Do what you are told by your boss.
Keep your mouth shut, no matter what.
No one talks to the cops, ever.
Even if that means going to jail.
Protect women and children.[9]
Severely punish anyone who hurts women and children.

Step up and take a beating when you deserve it.
Step up and give a beating when you need to.[10]
Always back your crew.

TERRY, JAIL, 2011

Terry had numerous cuts and bruises on his face and arms when he walked into the field office in the late summer of 2011. Nevertheless, he seemed to be in good spirits and looking forward to our outing. Our plan was to travel by SkyTrain out to the suburb of Delta to take photographs of the neighborhood where he grew up before entering the foster care system at age eleven. Terry's photo essay centered on the places of his childhood, which he imagined finding his way back to. He longed to reconnect with his family, who had adopted him when he was two years old. He often told me over the years that their unconditional support would motivate him to quit using drugs and doing crime for good. Many of those I knew went to great lengths not to think about the past. Terry, however, seemed to like looking back on an idealized childhood that was a stark contrast to the more painful aspects of his present.

In 2011 Terry was allowed to visit his childhood home only for Sunday dinners followed by a movie night. He would often ride his BMX bike all the way from downtown Vancouver to Delta to attend these weekly family gatherings, carefully tinkering with licit and illicit substances to get perfectly level for the occasion. Even once he was no longer allowed to enter his childhood home, Terry remained close with his grandma, who also lived in Delta. While she would also not permit Terry to live with her, she did collect the rent portion of his disability welfare check at her address and invited him over once a month or whenever he was released from jail so that he could pick up his money and enjoy a home-cooked meal and shower.

Prior to the summer of 2011, I had not seen Terry in over six months. I knew that he must have been in jail again. He confirmed this when I finally ran into him near one of his regular sleeping spots underneath a Shopper's Drug Mart overhang, just a few blocks from the field office. Ironically, the Shopper's Drug Mart that he was sleeping outside of was the same one where he had been arrested eight months earlier for shoplifting over three hundred dollars' worth of merch. Terry and a number of others were banned from entering this large drug store and had to wait outside whenever I went in to purchase the disposable cameras that we sometimes used for their photography projects. They were, however, generally permitted to sleep underneath the overhang or in a small alcove on the side of the building. They used flattened cardboard and wooden crates fished out of one of the large industrial bins behind the store to pad the ground and erect makeshift shelters. Upon running into Terry in his sleeping spot, we made plans to continue the photo essay project together the following week by heading out to Delta to take photographs.

Terry and a number of the other young men I knew were constantly in and out of jail for periods ranging from a few days to more than a year. While young people of all genders could become involved in low-level, loosely gang-connected dealing and other forms of crime, it was primarily the young men I knew who became more seriously embroiled in these activities, which almost inevitably led to jail time.[11] This time Terry landed in jail on shoplifting charges and for breaking the conditions of his parole, but he had a long history of serving longer sentences related to dealing, robbery, and theft.

Sometimes, Terry sent me letters from jail. They often featured stories from his childhood. One detailed his initiation into gang-connected crime at age thirteen, which he recalled as simultaneously exhilarating and terrifying:

Hi Danya how are you I'm fine thankz. I am sorry I was unable to be @ your office monday But I've Been in Jail since Thursday night. I'm locked up once again. I missed a probation appointment and found myself on the wrong side of the LAW. Oh well. Should be out in less than a month gonna get 2-4-1 days [serve half the time] because I'm in segregation 23 hour lockdown due to overflow in the Jails. they've got no more Room here.

I'm gonna try & write that diary I told you about in my last letter. I'm gonna write about previous days/weeks/months/years in my life and I'm also gonna write some pages on days that are happening as we speak. I'm hoping it comes in handy in your Project 4 UBC & I'm hoping some of the info will go in your Book. Included in this letter is a page that covers two or three days that took place over a week about 5–6 years ago. While I was wasting away in a foster house. It was a lot of fun But this was about the time my life flipped & turned upside down. this time would change the course of my life & this is where stuff goes haywire.

A Short Story By: T. B. L. ©
Life in The Fast Lane:
    Darren knocked on my door. I opened it he said, ah wanna Jack a Ride [steal a car]? Hell yeah! Oh man! Its fun as hell. So what do you think can I Parallel park this car @ 100 mph screech rrr screeeech perfect. Told ya I'd Been Practicing never had a license But I'd chase most pros off the track in seconds. Doin burnouts, drivin around. High speed chase getting away from the cops. It was Awesome.

That's how it started it was f-ckin scary. I thought I'm gonna to die. It was like shooting heroin, snorting coke & smoking a Joint one after the other while on the world's scariest roller coaster. the beginning of a long long love—hate Relationship. They [gang members] said Yeah, hell have a gun. Pull it. Five grand later and one less hater.

There is always work. When it's not Legit you Just create Your own. Make—money—Take—money. "Hard work the only kind of work that works" ⇐ a line from a movie

The story in Terry's letter was a continuation of one he had told me during one of our first conversations in 2008. "The foster care home was really, uh"—he searched for the word—"*menacing*? Everything was too lenient, so we took advantage all the time. We ended up going out at night to do stuff like, um, stealing cars, doing robberies. [Gang members] would just show up at the foster house, right? In their nicest clothes, with their nicest cars, stuff like that. It would always be when they had a bunch of money, eh? They'd have like two grand in their pocket and they'd want to make some more money out of it. So they'd come to us and they'd be like, enticing you to do it, like, 'I'll give you like five hundred bucks right now, but next week you gotta bring me a [stolen] car.' And that's how I got hooked up with those people. They came over to the foster house. They partied with us. They drank with us. They had all the money and ran the show."

"In some ways it's the time of our lives, right?" Terry mused. "It was so—um—*exciting*. It brought out the best and the worst in us. Like, I didn't use hard drugs back then, because they [gang members] will beat the *shit* out of you if they see you really messing up with drugs, right? So, I was just having *fun* at that point. God, *so* much fun. Drinking, partying, buying nice clothes! I was robbing [cannabis] grow-ops. Like, people were hiring us to rob gang members' grow-ops. Breaking into houses, climbing balconies. They like people who are young to do that stuff, because you don't get busted [go to jail], really." As he said this, it struck me that Terry's own experiences of cycling in and out of juvenile and adult criminal justice facilities throughout his entire adolescence and young adulthood seemed to belie this statement, even if the sentences he had served when he was younger were more lenient.

He continued, "And, these guys, like—they're, like, kind of a father figure, or a big brother. It's, like, a really messed up family. That protects you. That takes care of you. But that also gets you into so much trouble." He paused. "But the whole time I was with them, and doing that stuff, I remember I had this really vivid image in my head that I was going to die—like I could picture it *exactly*, how it would happen. I would get stabbed in the stomach and just left there alone on the sidewalk to die."

I first met Terry in 2008. Between 2008 and 2009, he spent time at the Lighthouse shelter. His stays were always brief, however, and over the years he returned again and again to sleeping outside, even as government-subsidized housing became increasingly available. One reason for this was the additional monthly income that he could generate by having his grandma collect the rent portion of his disability welfare check, rather than having this automatically allotted to social housing. Another reason was his frequent incarceration, which constantly thwarted his ability to stay anywhere for long.

When I met him in 2008, Terry had only recently become homeless in the city. For two years prior to that, he had been living in an apartment complex in Burnaby, which one of his foster fathers had helped him to secure as part of a Youth Agreement when he was sixteen. This legal agreement with the Ministry of Children and Family Development allows young people to live independently as emancipated minors, provided they meet certain obligations, such as working toward school completion and maintaining steady employment. While Terry had been initiated into gang-connected crime when he was thirteen, for years he moved between legal and illegal work. When he was fifteen, for example, he hopped a train to a city in the interior of BC and found temporary work on various construction sites. Upon returning to Vancouver when he was sixteen, he secured work with a local contracting company, also with the help of his foster father. Terry spent the next year and a half working on the construction of new Boston Pizza locations all over Greater Vancouver. Working these jobs meant that he had money to spend in the drug scenes that exist on the peripheries of construction industries across the province, and his use of alcohol, crack, and powder cocaine slowly intensified. At a certain point a friend from one of his old group homes unofficially moved into his apartment in Burnaby. Through the gang connections the two of them had established while in government care, they began dealing drugs from the apartment. Terry also continued to steal the odd car for profit.

He recalled in 2008, "We had *a lot* of drugs. Had *lots* of money. I had everything I could want and need in my house. I had a TV! I had a stereo! At one point I had five stereos in our place and I didn't even listen to all of them. They were just sitting on the floor! Had TVs in all the rooms. Had my bear sprays, all the weapons I needed in case anyone tried to mess with us, right? Man. I had video games. I was always drinking, partying *every night*—you know, call a group of friends over. Have like fifteen people in my house and have a bunch of beer and weed. It was the greatest time."

Eventually, Terry began doing more and more of his own product, including heroin. His roommate saw the writing on the wall and moved out. Between the loss of his roommate and business partner and the growing intensity of his own substance use, Terry could not continue dealing drugs at the same volume. Eventually he was kicked out of the apartment for causing damage to the property and found himself homeless. He then relocated to downtown Vancouver.

Even in 2011, after he had been homeless in Vancouver for almost four years, Terry loved to reminisce at length about his earlier life. He talked often about how involvement in gang-connected dealing and crime had made him feel untouchable and on top of the world for the first time in his life. It had also been a way into more "normal" dreams of place, such as having a girlfriend from a "good" family.

"I've driven Mercedes, Acuras, Range Rovers, you name it," he boasted that day as we sped out toward Delta on the SkyTrain. "Been in every [night]club in Vancouver pretty much, even though I was *way* too young to be in there, right? I used to order the most *expensive* stuff on the menu—don't even really know what I drank, eh? But I just know it was the most expensive, and had names I couldn't pronounce. And I bought clothes! Nice clothes and jewelry. I used to wear these, like, really colorful suits that cost like three hundred bucks a pop! I even had a good, *normal* girlfriend," he sighed. "Her dad was a *doctor*. She lived in a beach house four blocks from where my parents live. She had a golden retriever, and we used to take it for walks on the beach."

Gang-connected dealing and crime allowed Terry and many others to make money, assert hierarchies, wield reputations, and orchestrate various achievements and defeats with an intensity—a sense of momentum—that was not possible for them in the legal economy. It opened up forms of belonging and becoming in the City of Vancouver that were deeply desired and brought young people into the places that "normal rich kids" (as another young man I knew once put it) had access to, such as nice apartments and designer clothing stores—for a time, at least.

During the first few years of our acquaintance, Terry still had a few treasured items of clothing and jewelry that he had procured when he was making good money dealing, stealing cars, and doing crime. Often when we saw each other he would be conspicuously dressed in embellished Ed Hardy–style T-shirts, jeans, and hats. Across this period, Terry continued to deal drugs—albeit on a much smaller scale—whenever possible. He continued to have various gang-connected hookups from his past who would supply him with anywhere from fifty to two hundred dollars' worth of cannabis or heroin (and later fentanyl). On Welfare Wednesdays when Terry had extra cash, he often traveled by SkyTrain out to one such dealer's residence where he could get a particularly good price. Terry broke down however much he was able to afford (and manage to return to downtown Vancouver with) into ten-dollar flaps to sell along Granville and Hastings streets. When it came to this kind of street-level drug dealing, the Downtown Eastside in particular was viewed as an equal opportunity employer.

"Hastings is Hastings," Terry said to me on one occasion as we were walking through the neighborhood. "The police don't give a *shit* what happens here," he smirked, gesturing vaguely at a buzzing congregation of dealers and users on one street corner. "Anyone can sell dope just about anywhere they want. There are only a few corners that are owned turf [controlled by a gang]. So a lot of the rules that, like, apply *big time* when you are working for gangs don't actually really apply down here."

The fact that street-level dealing was largely permitted in the Downtown Eastside at this time was, in many moments, celebrated by young people as a frontier of economic opportunity in the margins (Roitman 2005), in which anyone could legitimately stake a claim and potentially get ahead in the city. In other moments, however, this leniency fueled the symbolic violence of ending up in the neighborhood. Those I followed did not generally embrace the image of Vancouver as the site of world-class progressive drug policies in straightforward ways. In many moments they expressed markedly conservative views regarding the need to crack down on open drug use in the city and in the Downtown Eastside in particular. Relaxed policing was read by some as evidence that "normal" people didn't care about what happened down there, further underscoring the marginality of the neighborhood and the extent to which it was a glaring exception to the politics of place that existed in "nicer" parts of Vancouver. This marginality was only compounded by the fact that strictly enforced moral logics of the gang also seemed to be largely absent from the Hastings corridor.

"Everyone down here tries to be a baller [player in the drug-dealing game] on Welfare Day," Terry explained that day in the Downtown Eastside. "People think, woo hoo, I got this much money. I'm gonna buy five hundred dollars' worth of drugs and sell it all and then I'll *always* have money and drugs. But no one ever does it. The next day everyone's on the grind. 'Oh, can I front [borrow] ten bucks?' Blah, blah, blah. Everyone's broke or in debt."

This was a pattern that Terry himself seemed to repeat month after month, although he always insisted that his aspirations were much grander and talked about saving money for a "real" (i.e., not government-subsidized) apartment in the city and a motorbike. In addition to regularly accruing drug debts, Terry's propensity for stretching the larger quantities of drugs he was able to procure on some Welfare Days into as many ten-dollar flaps as possible also often got him into trouble. One of these was the likely cause of the cuts and bruises that he had that day in the late summer of 2011. But whenever I talked to him about these dynamics and associated forms of violence, Terry seemed unperturbed, dismissive even. That was the game, he told me. And even those moments when things went off the rails were charged with possibility.

"Mentally, dealing—and even, like, debts—all of that shit, right? It's kind of *challenging*," he said that day on the SkyTrain in 2011. "Which is good. You have to keep six [watch out for police] all the time—oh shit, there's a cop walking by, but I got whatever amount on me, right? What do I do? Right? Like, oh shit, that guy's after me [over a debt or because of being ripped off], right? How do I fix that? What do I gotta do today to try and *get ahead*, right? It's challenging, but like, it's not so hard that I can't do it. It's fun. It's actually just fun. And, like, without that, it's almost like, what else is there?"

By 2011, Terry and many other young men I knew were as likely to go to jail on shoplifting charges as for dealing or other kinds of crime. Terry spent his days moving across Greater Vancouver, shoplifting merch from large shopping malls and big-box grocery, drug, and liquor stores. The huge quantities of cheese, meat, healthcare and beauty products, and clothing that he lifted could usually be traded for drugs, provided there was a dealer interested in the specific items he had procured (indeed, it was striking to enter the homes of these dealers and find them packed full of merch, the fridge loaded up with T-bone steaks, prime rib, and large blocks of cheese).

Terry was no longer untouchable—if that had indeed ever been the case—and on top of the world. When he was not in jail, he spent most of his nights sleeping outside. And yet it seemed to me that his life continued to be powerfully animated by the moral—if not material—worlds of the gang. While we were together, he frequently became caught up in the lively telling and retelling of stories about doing crime, getting away with it or getting arrested, going to court, and spending time in jail, always with a focus on the lessons about right and wrong that should follow from these accounts. Terry's stories could veer into more fantastical accounts of kidnappings, beatings, and even killings that he had heard about or been peripherally involved in. Some sounded like they could be true; others seemed to incorporate elements of the plotlines of popular gangster films. Terry told me these stories again and again while simultaneously concluding on several occasions that involvement in gang-connected crime and repeated incarcerations had ultimately caused his life to collapse. Like so many others, he was alternatively elated and haunted by the violence that he had witnessed and perpetrated (Fast, Shoveller, and Kerr 2017; Karandinos et al. 2014). He admitted to me more than once that he had never been able to shed the sense that he was about to die. He had a pain in his stomach that he imagined felt exactly like being stabbed.

On the SkyTrain that day in 2011, after listening to yet another a raucous story about the time that Terry and his buddy were in court and began harassing the bailiff by throwing gang signs, I asked him, "It's not all fun though, right? I mean, there are hard things about going to court over and over, and to jail again and again. Right?" I was trying, rather clumsily, to lead him to an answer I felt sure was there, which focused on the harms of repeated incarcerations. I had of course seen him experience many of these harms, such as repeated periods of street-based homelessness and the increased number of infections and other illnesses that tended to accompany them.

Terry had to compose himself before continuing. He was still laughing at the memory of how he and his friend had to be escorted out of the courthouse and their court date reset with a new bailiff. "You know, I've probably been to court *forty or fifty times*," he said finally. "Jail just appeared one day at my doorstep and said welcome home, sir!" I noticed several people in the SkyTrain car sneak glances in our direction. Terry made no effort to lower his voice. "But jail's not so bad, though, you know? There's a *pride* to being inside, right? There's *respect* that you get, from the other guys who are in there. For doing your time. For keeping your mouth shut." It struck me that the last few times he had been to jail it had seemed to have nothing to do with keeping his mouth shut and taking a charge for a higher-level boss. But that detail seemed unimportant to the story he was telling and the affective intensity that it was generating.

He continued, "And when you do get out—god, it's the greatest feeling in the world! You're all *refreshed* and ready to go. Straight back to the block [to deal drugs], with money in my pocket because my welfare checks are waiting for me [at his grandma's house]. Every time I go to jail, it's like—not a *vacation*, but, like— gain some weight, get healthy. Especially if you get two years plus a day," he added earnestly. "If you get under two years you go to provincial [jail]. But if you get two years plus a day you go to federal [jail] and you get all these programs. You can go to AA [Alcoholics Anonymous]. You can go to church. You can go to welding class."

For most of the young men I knew experiences and understandings of incarceration were complex. Cycling in and out of jail powerfully intersected a sense of getting lost and going nowhere in the city. Jail could be just one more in a long line of places where young people found themselves sinking into stagnation. It could be a continuation of the social suffering they had experienced across time and place and yet also, for some, an amelioration of that suffering. A number confided to me that a part of them *wanted* to be in jail. Given the chronic violence and instability they experienced outside, the structured routines of incarceration were comforting. Moreover, jail could be the site of exhilarating forms of sociality and magnetizing moral worlds of the gang, which generated a sense of momentum and possibility while inside and upon release.

"God, I wish I'd gone to school though!" Terry added suddenly as we neared our stop. "I missed prom. I missed all that shit. I always wanted to bring the nicest looking girl to prom. Or if she wasn't the nicest looking girl, she was *my* girl." He let out a long sigh, suddenly deflated of all his previous bravado. It seemed that the material and moral worlds of gang-connected dealing and crime had not been a way into all of Terry's dreams of place after all, even if they had, for a time, been a way into some of them. He was a shrewd hustler who had, for a time at least, been able to access desirable places, things, and status in the city. But he was also a kid who longed to go to high school and have a girlfriend whom he could take to the prom.

CARLY AND CONNOR, APARTMENT, 2013

In early 2013 Carly and Connor managed to secure a market rental apartment in a residential neighborhood in the south of Vancouver. I visited them shortly after they had moved in, laden with bags of secondhand housewarming gifts that I had started collecting as soon as I heard the news about their new place. Carly came down to the front door of the building to let me in since they did not yet have their buzzer set up. She was wearing a large purple fuzzy robe and pair of oversized cartoon character slippers, her hair still wet from the shower. As we rode the elevator to the fourth floor, Carly told me that she had been battling a piercing migraine all day and was not feeling well. Nevertheless, entering the new apartment felt like a momentous occasion. Carly had worked so hard to secure this place where she and Connor hoped to finally make a home with their two daughters. They had a new, more sympathetic social worker who had helped Carly to secure some government child benefit money so that she could afford the rent and damage deposit.

The smell of stale cigarette smoke was immediate as we entered the apartment, but it was bright and reasonably spacious. Carly collapsed back onto a large brown couch to continue watching daytime soap operas on TV while Connor jumped up to give me a tour. In the single bedroom a mattress was neatly made up with bedding and a carefully folded homemade quilt. A bedside table towered somewhat awkwardly above the mattress because they did not yet have a bed frame. On it were three framed photographs of Carly and Connor with their second daughter, taken at the hospital just one day after she was born. In the kitchen, Connor showed me inside each and every cupboard. Boxes of cereal and pasta were meticulously arranged into a fan so that the front of each product was visible. Various dishware was perfectly placed in neat rows. I felt certain that they must have been anticipating an inspection by their social workers at any moment; my tour of the apartment felt like a dress rehearsal.

"Carly is really trying to lose weight right now," Connor said, gesturing at the produce drawer in the fridge full of fruits and vegetables and at the bottles of Hydroxycut and other vitamins that lined the top of the kitchen stove. "Right, Carly?" he asked pointedly. He seemed annoyed by her low energy. Meanwhile, he was buzzing, moving rapidly from drawer to drawer to show me every cooking utensil and dishcloth.

"Yeah," Carly said. "I am. I've already lost, like, fifteen pounds actually. And Connor is supposed to be looking into going back to treatment," she shot back. "Aren't you?"

"I'm not the only one who left treatment, Carly," Connor said, his voice rising. "Just remember that you left, too."

Carly and Connor had secured this apartment and filled it with all of the things they needed, which was a condition of regaining custody of their daughters. However, neither had yet fulfilled another of the social worker's demands: namely, that each attend a separate residential treatment program and demonstrate that they were actively working on their recovery.

"I did leave my program," Carly admitted, turning to look at me. "I honestly *hated* it at the place that I was at, and I also just know that I don't, like, *need* treatment. Like, our issue has always been *housing*. I've always said, if I have housing, I will stop using. And I am *not* using at the moment, right?"

"What did you hate about the treatment place?" I asked.

Carly launched into a long story about how the staff had unfairly accused her of trying to bring "unauthorized opioids" into the treatment center and denied her legitimate prescription pain medications. By the end of the story, it sounded to me like she might have been kicked out of the center, rather than having left on her own initiative. Connor then launched into his own long story about how he had left his residential program after an irritating altercation with another resident that he had ultimately not been willing to work through with the program staff.

I frequently observed that the moral worlds young people spent so much time elaborating, embodying, and defending on the streets often followed them into residential treatment with disastrous results. On the streets, accusations and altercations of the kind that both Carly and Connor had experienced while in treatment almost always escalated into full-blown dramas that then had to be resolved with loud and violent confrontations. Or they were not resolved at all; young people frequently broke off relationships with former romantic partners, friends, and chosen family members, vowing to never again have anything to do with them. This kind of escalation and drama was largely unacceptable in the residential treatment centers where I spent time, and I watched as individuals got kicked out or left again and again. The thing that engendered a valued sense of momentum and being at the center of something on the streets often produced stalls and dead ends in young people's treatment trajectories.

Beyond the drama that had occurred at each of their residential treatment centers, Carly and Connor were not willing to separate from each other for the three- to six-month period required by their respective residential treatment programs. They were certain that what was right was for them to stay together as they attempted to create a home and family with their daughters.

"They are trying to isolate us from each other, when we know that we *need* to stay together no matter what," Carly said that day in her new apartment. "We are only going to succeed together. Two—uh—brains is better than one, right?"

"They [social workers] don't understand that," Connor cut in. "They think that being apart and focusing on yourself, *that's* what works. But it doesn't. People need each other, right? Like, without each other? We *really* have nothing. At least until my kids are back with me."

Less than a year after this visit to their apartment, Carly and Connor permanently lost custody of their two daughters. A few months before they received the court's decision, they both relapsed on crack. Connor, perhaps, had never really stopped using. But my sense was that it was Connor's worsening schizophrenia and a violent incident that had occurred between him and Carly at the apartment, which landed Connor in jail, that ultimately raised the alarm and resulted in permanent custody loss.

Carly and Connor were devastated by this outcome. They were also deeply, painfully exhausted. From their perspective, they had worked hard to do every single thing that the social workers had asked of them, while maintaining their fierce commitment to each other and their dream of creating a family together. And now, despite all that work, they were left with nothing except the terrible, irredeemable loss of their daughters. A week after they had lost custody, Carly told me tearfully that the loss she felt had been made that much worse by the fact that the social workers and other professionals had seemed to string them along for so long, when in fact they had never had a hope of getting their kids back.

"We did this, we did that. We ran all over this city, from this meeting to that meeting. We got the *apartment*. Got all the stuff in it for our girls to come home. The only thing we didn't do is give up each other." She paused to compose herself. "Which, like, I still stand behind my decision to stay with Connor. Because it's like—do you want us to have *nothing at all* in our lives? Like, how can they ask us to have *nothing* while we are working on these things, right? Like, without each other, we can't keep ourselves *going* with all of the shit that they are asking of us." After a while, she added, "I mean, I guess in the end maybe we couldn't keep going—couldn't, like, hold it all together—even with each other's support. It was just too hard."

STAGNATION

Even as addiction, romantic relationships, drug dealing, debts, and crime generated significant momentum and possibility in young people's day-to-day lives, the threat of stagnation loomed constantly. Many I knew seemed to oscillate between a sense of being at the center of something rife with potential and a sense that they were stuck, trapped, and going nowhere. An affective sense of stagnation was often expressed through the language of boredom, a remarkably common vocabulary of discontent among those I followed. Far more often than young people questioned why I would want to put myself in potentially risky situations in order to do this research, they remarked on how boring it must be for me to hang around with them, "killing time" (Bengtsson 2012; Ralph 2008). They used the language of boredom to explain why they had left the places of their childhoods and ended up in Vancouver ("I was just so bored at my group home"), why they transitioned from one substance to another ("I get bored of one drug and I move on to the next"), and why they wanted to leave drug scene involvement behind ("I want to go back to school and get a job, because it's so boring out here"). They also used the language of boredom to explain why, even after exiting Greater Vancouver's drug scenes for a period, they found themselves reentering them periodically as a way of regaining a desired sense of forward momentum in their lives ("When you're out of it, there are no extremes. There's no nothing. There's no bad, but there's no good either").

JANET, TRAFALGAR HOTEL, 2010

"I haven't left this place in a year," Janet said in 2010. "I'm bored out of my mind by all of this shit. Boring, boring, boring, bored, bored, bored, bored." We were standing in the hallway outside her room in the Trafalgar Hotel, which always seemed to be full of people in various states of coming up and coming down off drugs. The skin around Janet's left eye was bruised and swollen. She told me her boyfriend had jealousy issues and some of her dates could be psychos. She did not specify which had been the cause of her black eye. She looked tired. "I need to get the f-ck out of here," she mumbled, almost inaudibly, as she slid down the wall to sit on the dirty floor of the hallway.

PATTY AND JOE, MACKENZIE HOTEL, 2010

While we were sitting in her room at the Mackenzie Hotel in 2010, Patty told me that she wished she could go back in time and tell herself never to come to Vancouver. She had been talking to me again about her hep C diagnosis, which continued to devastate her. She said she felt ruined.

"And it's just, like, so hard to live a *normal* life here," she said. "There's not much work here at all. Like, I've *had* jobs, back in Edmonton. Laboring jobs for a roofing company, construction companies—temp agency stuff. Dish-washing jobs. I've worked at convenience stores, fast-food joints. Lots of stuff, yeah. But here, like, I haven't really been able to do any of that."

Patty had recently been evicted from the Trafalgar Hotel, where she and Joe had both been moved after the Lighthouse shelter was shut down. Joe was still technically living at the Trafalgar. However, Patty was sneaking him into the Mackenzie as often as she could, risking yet another eviction. She was irate that the building managers at both the Mackenzie and the Trafalgar seemed determined to split her and Joe apart, when everything that was happening in their world told them how important it was for them to stay together.

During this period, evictions from hotels like the Mackenzie and the Trafalgar and other similar places were extremely common. Young people were usually evicted for breaking visitor policies (whether to broker drug deals or sleep in the same place as their romantic partners) and for noise complaints (usually as a result of drug deals or romantic relationships gone wrong). When evictions occurred, many found themselves with nowhere to go. Particularly toward the beginning of this project, evictions and periods of hospitalization and incarceration were almost always followed up with periods of street-based homelessness. Other young people were quickly put into another SRO managed by the same social housing agency (as Patty had been when she was moved from the Trafalgar to the Mackenzie)—where most eventually faced yet another eviction, and so on.

"There's a lot more informal work here though, hey?" Joe replied, somewhat uncharacteristically. When he, Patty, and I were together, Patty did most of the talking. "Everybody here drug deals and does crime and stuff."

"But one minute there's people that are, like, big time, and then the next minute they're thrown in jail," Patty said. "And then there's somebody else who takes over [that drug-dealing turf] right away, so." Neither she nor Joe had ever seemed to show much interest in dealing. In 2010, they were primarily relying on their monthly social assistance checks and trading and selling shoplifted merch to generate income.

"There's lots of services here, though," Patty acknowledged diplomatically. "That's pretty much what takes up all our time, now. Trying to figure out where to eat and trying to figure out, like, what to do to—like, get Joe on disability welfare, try to figure out where to get a resume done and get clean clothes and look into school, like—it takes up so much of your time when you're homeless, just, like, all of that stuff. It's just kind of a circle—cycle—that you get stuck in." I found it interesting that Patty continued to refer to herself as homeless, even though she had technically been housed for almost a year.

"But that's the way that we, like, need to fill our time. Especially right now," she said. "It's a pretty boring life, at the moment. But me and Joe are trying to do things a bit different, at the moment." Patty and Joe had recently made the decision to quit doing sex work (although it seemed to me that Patty had largely made the decision). They never provided me with much in the way of an explanation for this shift. I knew that both had experienced violent encounters with dates over the years and that Patty worried constantly about Joe's physical, psychological, and emotional well-being. Also during this period, however, Patty had completed an assessment related to getting her GED and was ecstatic when the results had revealed that she had a twelfth grade reading level. She had started talking to me about returning to school. On several occasions we pored over an increasingly battered course catalogue together so that we could discuss what she might like to take to meet the GED requirements.

"These days, I can't stand weekends," Patty continued.

"That's interesting," I replied. "Cause that's sort of the opposite of what you would say if—"

"—if you worked," she interrupted, laughing. "If you had a normal life. But for people like us, we usually can't stand the weekends. Everything is closed. So we can't, like, make progress on anything. We can't fill our days, you know?"

ENDLESS BUSINESS

Among young people, time was often marked by elaborate itineraries associated with the drama of the local drug scenes. It was also marked by a seemingly endless process of collating and checking off items on one's to-do list:

Apply for government identification.
Apply for an Indian Status Card.
Apply for a Social Insurance Number.
Make a resume.
Apply for school.
Apply for training programs.
Apply for jobs.
Find a shelter.
Find social housing.
Find better social housing.
Fill out the forms to get better social housing.
Make phone calls related to getting better social housing.
Get on welfare.
Get on better, disability welfare.
Get on methadone.
Get back on methadone.
Go to court.
Go stand in food, shower, and laundry lines.
Go to appointments.

This endless round of business (Preble and Casey 1969) structured young people's time in ways that were perhaps preferable to sitting around with nothing to do. However, unlike the drama of the scene, the itineraries generated by the care assemblage seemed to discipline time in such a way that could render each moment the same (Musharbash 2007). Enmeshed in the rhythms and routines of the public health and poverty management infrastructures, "the present [could become] oppressive, like a cage in which one [was] caught, in which one experience[d] the same thing over and over again" (Musharbash 2007, 313). The result was a crushing, painful sense of boredom, even as young people attempted to make various kinds of progress. In response, those I followed were drawn again and again toward particular kinds of escapes and flights via drug use, dealing, debts, crime, and new romantic relationships and business partnerships. Stagnation contained an imperative for action (Brissett and Snow 1993). Alternatively, they stayed in their rooms—sometimes for weeks on end—spending vast amounts of time doing drugs, sleeping, and binge-watching TV. But it seemed that even the fun of "getting into trouble" (Jervis, Spicer, and Manson 2003) and pleasurable forms of suspension could become boring, particularly for those who longed to structure their time around work, school, and domestic routines. In the absence of meaningful markers of time, young people frequently expressed a sense of stagnation, even in the midst of chaos (Brissett and Snow 1993).

TERRY, FIELD OFFICE, 2012

"I'm really getting somewhere with this now, I think," Terry said, referring to our collaboration on this research project, which was perhaps just one more item in the endless round of business young people were contending with. "I think that this could actually take me places!"

LEE, MACKENZIE HOTEL, 2012

"I want to get ahead here," Lee told me in 2012. "I want to progress." He tried to sound confident but grew increasingly agitated as he shuffled through a stack of photographs he had taken one year earlier. We were standing outside the Mackenzie Hotel, trying to decide where to go next. Lee never invited me into his building, even though I ran into him frequently while spending time there with other individuals.

Lee and many others struggled to reconcile their entrenched social, spatial, and economic exclusion in the city with their desires to situate themselves as a part of it. The process of reflecting back on our time together as my doctoral program drew to a close in 2012 could be painful for many. As I passed this significant milestone, those who were a part of my research often reflected with deep sadness that they were nowhere near where they thought they would be when we first met.

Nevertheless, Lee perhaps more so than others I knew looked again and again to the possibilities of an ever-evolving array of state-sponsored programs and services in order to make changes in the trajectory of his life. Lee's life had been torn apart by his time in government care. As he said to me in 2010, being removed from his family and cycling between government foster care and group homes caused everything to "explode," and he had been attempting to put the pieces back together ever since. Lee often fondly recalled one of the group homes that he had stayed in as an adolescent, which provided a period of stability. He remembered the volunteer work that he had done at a local farm as part of the programming there and how one of the staff members had helped him to secure work at a local fast-food restaurant. Perhaps these memories partially explained his ongoing belief that services and systems might eventually provide a way forward, a way out of his current circumstances.

Despite the ways in which the state had failed him, he continued to throw himself into the endless round of business created by the poverty management and public health infrastructures in downtown Vancouver. Without fail, whenever we saw each other, he always took time to list the maze of services, agencies, and bureaucracies that he was navigating.

"There's these new programs now—or whatever—down here," he said vaguely that day in 2012, as we walked toward a fast-food restaurant. "You can become whatever you want I guess—that's what [the program staff] said? They're like, yeah, pretty much whatever you want cause there's so much demand for workers?" He sounded unsure. "So, I have to get my resume ready, get my [government] ID, get my Indian status card. And I'm trying to get a new place to stay. Last night my [SRO] door got kicked in for no good reason, just people being crazy. I need to call the [social housing agency] today."

Lee also looked beyond the care assemblage for ways to put his life back together. He longed to reconnect with aspects of his Indigenous identity and attended as many free cultural events in the city as possible. In 2012 he invited me to come with him and some other friends to a large National Indigenous People's Day celebration in a local park. We camped out on a spot on the grass for hours, eating and drinking and enjoying the musical performances and speeches. Lee and his friends darted off every so often to use drugs and became progressively more high and drunk as the afternoon progressed. Lee looked to meth to get him going, to keep him moving forward, and to "get him out of a boring state," as he once put it. Between 2012 and 2015 he oscillated between trying to avoid meth, crack, and alcohol and falling into periods of intensive use that also coincided with time spent in the "drunk tank" (a jail cell accommodating people who are intoxicated, usually with alcohol) and city jail. He told me he would wake up in both places with no memories of what had happened. Sometimes he had been beaten up or all of his possessions were gone.

Lee occasionally tried to make sense of these relapses through the language of peer pressure. Shortly after our time together at the National Indigenous People's Day celebration, he reflected, "My friends will be like, 'You want some?' And I'll say, 'No, man, I don't want any.' Or, like, 'I don't want any *more*.' But they'll be like, 'Keep on going, keep on going! Let's keep on going! Let's keep *this* going!' Right? And sometimes I *do* just want to keep it going, right?"

I had seen these kinds of encounters play out many times. It seemed, in some instances at least, that what was at stake was maintaining the intensity and momentum of the encounter and particular kinds of sociality in the context of looming stagnation, rather than what we might call peer pressure.

REENTERING NEVER NEVER LAND

Young people talked often about getting out: out of downtown, out of Greater Vancouver's various drug scenes, out of doing crime, and out of tumultuous relationships. Some turned to the poverty management and public health infrastructures to enact these escapes. Others attempted to do it on their own, usually by relocating.

On a number of occasions, I witnessed individuals pull themselves together in the ways that they often talked about: they went to treatment and got clean, moved into market rental apartments or basement suites or back in with family members, went back to school, and, very rarely, got part-time jobs (most continued to rely on social assistance, living with roommates to make ends meet in the absence of employment). I sat with them in sparsely decorated living rooms and kitchens as they attempted to place the new rhythms and routines of their lives within narratives of progress. They said that, eventually, they would get a better job. Eventually, they would have a career. Eventually, they would have the income to enjoy leisure activities in the evenings and on the weekends. But almost always they sounded uncertain and expressed a troubling sense that they were still somehow lost or going nowhere in the city. The changes in their lives weren't happening fast enough, and they continued to find themselves all too often sitting around with nothing to do. And they were more isolated now. There was no one around in the areas where they now lived. They never seemed to have any fun anymore. They felt sedated, numb, and very, very bored.

Unfortunately, young people's attempted exits often deepened a sense of stagnation rather than ameliorating it. They found themselves in situations in which there seemed to be nothing left to do except sit in their apartments or basement suites on welfare, where they were safe, perhaps, from risk but not from the structural violence of entrenched poverty and marginalization. Faced with this reality, many made the decision to reenter the fantasyland of Greater Vancouver's drug scenes. In certain moments the rapid succession of risks and rewards, constant problem solving, and frenetic sociality that characterized life on the streets—a sense of being at the center of something—seemed preferable to a sense that they were still, despite their efforts to do everything they were supposed to do, going nowhere. It was stressful, but it was better than nothing.

JORDAN, BEACHWOOD HOTEL, 2013

A few months after Jordan and I had gone to the community garden I ran into him on the street. He had his hood pulled up and dark sunglasses on, even though the sky was gray. He admitted that he had relapsed on heroin. But he was dressed that way, he told me, because of the hickeys on his neck and brutal hangover he was currently nursing. Last night he had hooked up again with a young woman who lived a few blocks away from him, and they had stayed up drinking.

As we walked together toward her building (Jordan said he was on his way to wake her up, even though it was three in the afternoon), he told me that he had started dealing drugs again. He had run into an old acquaintance with gang connections who had recently gotten out of jail and had access to a supply of heroin.

When Jordan proved over the course of two weeks that he could move some of this heroin "without messing up" (i.e., doing all of it himself and disappearing), he was quickly given more responsibility, including larger quantities of heroin to sell and oversight of two additional workers.

This was a pattern that would repeat itself over the next three years. When Jordan got clean, he imagined that he might never again be drawn back into the routines of drug use, crime, and care that seemed to trap him in the Downtown Eastside. After he relapsed, he usually commented to me that this was inevitable so long as he was living in an SRO in the neighborhood. It was just the way things were for "people like him" who "ended up" down there.

Only a half block away from his perhaps-girlfriend's SRO we ran into her dad, who informed us that she wasn't home. Jordan began pacing the sidewalk and cursing loudly, angrily insisting he had told her to wait for him at her building today. Her dad remained completely unphased and tight-lipped throughout all of this, coolly informing Jordan that he would tell her to meet him at *his* building later on. Jordan and I started walking back in that direction, him fuming the entire way but also expressing a sense of satisfaction that he would not have to share the drugs he had procured for both of them just prior to running into me. He invited me to come into his building, leading me up a flight of stairs to a shared lounge with two sagging couches and a plastic plant in the corner.

"I hate using. I hate drugs," he said as he prepared a syringe of heroin. "Drug using isn't normal. But honestly, I was just so bored. Right?"

He continued, "I'm actually *happier* now—now that I'm using again. When I'm sober I get into this mode where I just sit and sit and sit and sit and watch movies and TV. I get fat, just doing nothing. But now that I'm using and working from, uh, like seven A.M. to midnight? I've actually lost a bit of weight, recently. I'm moving around easier."

That was the thing: when Jordan and other young people I knew got clean, got jobs—often within the poverty management and public health infrastructure as "peer workers" or "peer researchers"—and even got out of downtown, the white picket fence life that so many of them dreamed of still wasn't remotely within reach. Instead, what they were met with were things like medication-assisted treatment and welfare checks and supportive housing. When he was clean and not doing crime, Jordan was safer and less at risk but also painfully bored. Rather than propelling him forward, the care assemblage engendered a sense of stagnation. Jordan could go for months without barely leaving his room, where he passed the time by watching endless episodes of *Law & Order*. Alternatively, he could be out on the streets, living out the more exciting aspects of the plotlines he saw repeated in loops on TV.

He reflected, "It's cooler now that I have to *work* for my dope. When I have to *work* for my high. The grind. When I got it for free [at the heroin maintenance trial], I didn't like it. It was like, man, I need to get *off* this shit. The crime is—it's a rush. I've got the best heroin on the block! And I'm a good worker, so the guy I know keeps giving me more and more responsibility with his product, right? And at least, down here, this is *something*. I'm good at it, right? I'm actually really good at all this," he chuckled. "And I'm free."

He went quiet, preparing to do his fix. I left him sitting there on the couch, staring out the window at the new condo units going up across the street.

The last time I saw Jordan was in late 2015. He came into the field office wearing a T-shirt and shorts even though it was freezing out. His eyes were half closed and a smile played on his lips. He was using heroin but had also gone back on methadone. He told me that he was taking methadone rather than returning to the heroin maintenance trial because he was certain that when that trial was over he would be left with no option but to take methadone anyways. "Why prolong the inevitable?" he said. "Programs like that always end."

Jordan was doing less dealing and crime and seemed to have sunk back into stagnation, which he largely attributed to the SRO where he was living. Violent incidents and break-ins to his room were constant. "I can't own anything nice," he said. "It will just get stolen."

Jordan told me that the previous year he had been on a waiting list for better government-subsidized housing and assured by workers that he would get a place soon. But recently he had had to start all over again to find a new place to live because his criminal record check had identified an assault charge from three years earlier, which meant that he was not currently eligible. Jordan became increasingly furious as he told me about how he was going to sue BC Housing for stringing him along. Those I knew often said things like this when their fragile sense of forward momentum and plans for the future were thwarted by the institutions that controlled various aspects of their lives. Threats of suing agencies, hospitals, and individuals seemed to be a way of momentarily regaining a sense of momentum when plans abruptly stalled, fell through, and dead-ended.

"I just spent the last year doing f-ck all," Jordan said. "Sitting in a room, waiting for them. Going back on methadone, doing less dope. Doing less crime. But it didn't make *any* difference to getting housing."

I asked him to say more about why he wasn't doing as much dealing and crime these days. I recalled how energized and happy he had been only a short time ago when he was heavily embroiled in both. "Are you afraid of going to jail?" I asked.

Jordan told me, not for the first time, that he both hated being institutionalized and longed for it—a tension that came up not infrequently with others too. Jordan had been incarcerated for much of his adolescence. He often described this period in positive terms. Incarceration was what got him away from an abusive, highly unstable family. It was what allowed him to complete some college-level courses. Sitting with me in the field office in 2015, he told me again that when he was finally released from jail at age seventeen he wasn't at all sure if he actually wanted to leave. "Like, I wanted to go back," Jordan said, and then added, "In a way, I still kind of do? In a way I'm scared of jail, and I don't want to go back to jail. But I do want to go back to jail."

"What is it about jail that makes you want to go back?" I asked.

"The seclusion, the-the-the—what's the word for that? Being confined to— just the daily *routine*. Every day's the same, being in jail. You *control* everything. I have to be able to control myself cause if I can't control myself it's like—" he didn't finish his sentence. While a feeling of being controlled inside jail sent some of those I knew into violent rages, Jordan longed for it, at least in certain moments. "Besides," he eventually added, "I'm already in jail. The way I live— my housing—I'm captive—it's—yeah." He trailed off again. Finally, he said, "I want to get out of here."

In that moment I wasn't sure if he meant the field office, his housing, or the City of Vancouver. I remained silent, waiting for him to elaborate. After a while he said, "Do you know what I'm going to do as soon as I get off methadone? I'm getting a camera, and I'm going up to northern Alaska and I'm going to move up into the wilderness. Get a bow and arrow. Go hunt. Build a cabin. If you home-stead on a place for six months, it can be yours," he said, shifting his posture so that he was sitting more upright. "Yeah. I plan on it as soon as I get off metha-done. Get my license, get a big four-door pickup truck, and drive me and my dog into the woods." Jordan had recently rescued a large huskie, whom he adored, from a friend. The dog was currently sitting at our feet, panting in the heat of the cramped room. "Can you get me a job?" he asked suddenly. "Up at UBC?"

Not for the first time I noticed that Jordan only seemed to be willing to live on the edge of certain kinds of changes: a "real" job, a "real" college or university education, a "real" adventure in the wilderness. He did not often seem willing to take the series of steps that would be required to get him into slightly better social housing or onto a better prescription opiate.

As our conversation drew to a close Jordan said, "If I'm going to die, I wanna go out and die in the wilderness." I knew that he had recently been diagnosed with cirrhosis of the liver, likely caused by hep C. "I don't wanna die down here," he told me.

But in the end, he never did leave Vancouver.

SHAE, MACKENZIE HOTEL, 2009

In the fall and winter of 2009 Shae stopped coming by to see me at the field office and messaging me on Facebook. I knew that they were living at the Mackenzie Hotel because Jeff had also been moved into the Mackenzie following the clo-sure of the Lighthouse; I visited him and Lula there often (although Lula was officially housed in a different building). But I never seemed to run into Shae there anymore. When Shae finally walked back into the field office at the end of December they looked horrible. I knew Shae to be energetic and charismatic, and that energy and charisma extended to their appearance. They favored tight, brightly colored T-shirts and jeans and often embellished their look with painted nails and flashy jewelry. That day, however, they appeared uncharacteristically gaunt and pale. Once we were seated together in a private room Shae told me through choking sobs that they had just called their mom to tell her that they were HIV-positive and that this was the first day they had left their room at the Mackenzie Hotel in over two months, when they had first learned of their diagnosis. They had spent most of that time sleeping, covering the windows in their room with tinfoil, and keeping the lights off for days on end, only opening the door a crack each day to indicate that they were still alive when the building manager or other staff came by for room checks. Shae said that many of their friends and chosen family had abandoned them, but a few people had occasionally brought them food from nearby meal programs. They had also brought heroin, which Shae began using.

Over the course of 2010 Shae slowly pulled themselves out of this period of depression, partially through the increasingly intensive use of meth, which also helped with getting off heroin (Fast et al. 2014). They began cycling through a number of SROs and supportive housing buildings as a result of evictions and building transfers. Eventually, in 2013, Shae was moved into Arbutus House, a newly built supportive housing building for individuals living with HIV. By this time Shae seemed to have made a certain amount of peace with their diagnosis. They were once again a fixture in the scene and an active and much-loved member of the gay and drag communities in Vancouver, performing under the name of their alter ego Trix. Yet over those years Shae talked to me often about their fear that they could at any moment be pulled under again, back into a state of crippling depression and intensive heroin use. This time, Shae said, the cause would not be a health crisis but rather the increasing isolation that they were contending with as a result of being progressively separated from the friends, family, and lovers who had once been allowed to stay together at the Lighthouse shelter and Mackenzie and Trafalgar hotels.

DISAPPEARANCES

As they attempted to make a place for themselves in the city, young people contended with the everyday and settler-colonial violence of various kinds of disappearances (Coulthard 2014; Tomiak 2019). There were many ways they could disappear for periods of time, including drug binges that kept them indoors somewhere or moving quickly from place to place for days on end. They frequently had to lay low and hide or keep moving to avoid being picked up by police for outstanding warrants and red zone violations or tracked down by friends, romantic partners, and associates to settle drug debts and other altercations. They were hospitalized for infections, overdoses, and periods of mental health crisis, went to jail, detox, and treatment, and were put into various supportive housing buildings.

There were also more permanent forms of disappearance. Stories circulated about individuals who were kidnapped and tortured and pushed out of SRO windows to their deaths. Overdoses could be fatal, including during the earliest years of my research. Several young people confided to me that they had attempted suicide in the past and sometimes still thought about dying. The line between suicide and overdose could be blurry (see also Garcia 2010). As the drug supply became increasingly adulterated with benzodiazepines in the later years of my research, periods of time increasingly disappeared from young people's memories, never to be recovered (Mullins 2022). Those witnessing these episodes commented that the people they knew and loved were disappearing right in front of them.

My research also overlapped with the Missing Women Commission of Inquiry, which began in 2010 and underscored the magnitude of police misconduct in response to the large number of women, particularly Indigenous women, who were reported missing from the Downtown Eastside in the late 1990s and early 2000s. What emerged from this inquiry was a confirmation of what many had long known—that reports of missing women had not been taken seriously by police because of the "kinds" of women involved (i.e., women who were engaged in sex work and drug use in the context of homelessness and unstable housing), leading to a large number of additional and preventable deaths. Many of these women are presumed dead at the hands of serial killer Robert Pickton (Oppal 2012). That these women had been forsaken (to use the language of the 2012 report from the inquiry) and allowed to disappear from the city haunted many of those I knew.

LEE, GONE, 2015

"I'm like—I'm stuck here," Lee said with frustration in 2013. We sat together in the park where he was currently sleeping, located behind St. Paul's Hospital. Sunlight filtered through the autumn leaves that still remained on the trees. "And I don't know what to do. I'm tired of this life, man. I'm *tired*. I don't love it. I *hate* it. Of course, I love the scenery, I love the city, but I hate what's in it—for myself, right?"

I had never heard Lee talk this way and wasn't quite sure what to say. I just sat there, listening.

He continued, "It's been, like, ten *years* since I moved here—just trying to live. Trying to not kill myself, you know what I mean? Trying to eat, trying to keep myself from—not going to jail or anything. I wish I had a job or I went to school. I try to—I try to stay busy, right?" He began reciting his usual to-do list: "I *got* to get my resume done. I know that I have to go to school—*finish* school. I've *got* to go to work. But sometimes you feel so worthless." He paused. "And you want to get help. *Help me* a little bit, right? Like, I wanna try—I wanna try and help myself but you gotta wait for the right housing and then if I did have housing I'd—God as my witness I would get my shit together. I would."

By this time, Lee was living in cleaner and safer supportive housing, but it was not the home he had imagined for himself. He continued to hold out hope that he would soon be offered nicer government-subsidized housing—a condominium in prime developments like the Olympic Village complex or renovated Woodward's building, for example.

"Have you been able to talk to someone about how you're feeling?" I asked, growing increasingly alarmed by how Lee was talking. In my mind I began going through the services and people I could connect Lee with that afternoon.

"Yeah. I've done it before," he replied, with little enthusiasm. "I've-I've-I've already done that, right? And, like, with all that, like, kind of stuff, it'll come back, like, uh, full circle. It's like I'm on a—uh—merry-go-round. Try to get help, try to get somewhere, but, like, come back again and again and again. *Same f-cking spot.*" He added, "And so then you do drugs you shouldn't do, and you drink even though you shouldn't be doing that, either, right? And you go around with people you shouldn't be [doing crime]—you know what I mean?"

Lee then told me that a friend of his had recently committed suicide. It had disturbed him deeply, he said, not just because of the loss but because the two of them had shared similar difficult circumstances. "What's the difference between how he was doing it and, like, the way I'm living?" Lee asked. "What's the difference? I'm still living with poverty. But it hasn't made *me* want to commit suicide." But then he added, "Maybe I'm *thinking* about killing myself sometimes, but I'm not going to do it. Am I stronger than him—than people who do that? That's the question."

After a while he added hopefully, "But, somebody told me that it's easy to die but it's harder—it's harder to live. I think it's a saying—people say that. And it's true. So, I'm going to keep trying—keep going. I have to. I have a lot of living to do."

We drank our coffees in silence for a while, until the sun dipped behind a building and it became too cold to sit in the park any longer.

Lee never was able to put his life back together in the ways that he dreamed of. He never did find the momentum he needed in the care assemblage of the state. I lost touch with Lee in mid-2014 and knew immediately that something was wrong. By 2015 rumors started circulating that he had been killed in a violent altercation at a halfway house. For a long time no one seemed able to determine what exactly had happened to Lee, including when he had moved out of his housing building and into the halfway house. Finally, I confirmed his death with a family member, although the details remained vague. Lee had disappeared. He was gone.

When I learned of his death I remembered the day several years earlier when we had driven together to Vancouver's North Shore Mountains. Lee had wanted to photograph the City of Vancouver from that vantage point for his photo essay, which was titled *Where I'm Going*. That day Lee had commented repeatedly on how at peace he felt, watching the views change out of the car window and then climbing over the rocks at Lighthouse Park, the city faintly visible on the horizon across a wide expanse of ocean. "I've never been this far *out* of downtown," he said softly at one point. "At least, not since I came to Vancouver. That's why I wanted to take this photograph—it's like a zoomed-out view of where I want to be. Like—you can't see any of the bad parts from here." He turned to look at me. "Thank you for taking me here."

Across the years I knew him Lee did not want to escape from the city. Quite the opposite. He longed for a place within it. However, from the vantage point of his supportive housing building or the various lines he stood in and appointments he attended daily, these dreams of place seemed increasingly out of reach. Toward the end of his life he questioned whether he could keep moving toward them. But sitting on the rocks of Lighthouse Park that day in 2012, gazing out across the ocean at the city, Lee saw, perhaps, what he continued to love about it.

PART 3

LOST

PATTY, CITY OF GLASS, 2011

"It seems like you aren't really *allowed* to be homeless in downtown Vancouver anymore," Patty joked half-heartedly in the summer of 2011. The sun beat down on the City of Glass, baking the concrete and steel of the downtown core and yellowing the grass of its public parks.[1] "No one is outside, anymore."

COMMUNITY CARE

The visibility of street-based homelessness in Vancouver's Downtown South has waxed and waned across time as political and economic forces continually remake the urban landscape. In 2008 and 2009, along Granville Street, groups of homeless young people could often be seen sitting in front of the string of restaurants, nightclubs, and retail stores that have gradually taken over the block, displaying handmade signs asking for money and food. At night they slept in the entryways and alcoves of these same establishments with blankets and sleeping bags pulled up over their heads, empty disposable coffee cups carefully set out beside them to collect donated change. By 2011 these bodies were much less visible on the sidewalks of the Downtown South. Where did they disappear to?

In the years leading up to and following the 2010 Winter Olympic Games, issues of visible homelessness, addiction, and related forms of "public disorder" in downtown Vancouver generated significant political, academic, and public attention (Stueck 2006). Under growing pressure to live up to promises made in Vancouver's successful 2002 Olympic bid and guided by the Vancouver Agreement's ethic of revitalization without displacement, in 2007 the city, provincial, and federal governments began spending millions of dollars to purchase over two dozen SROs in Vancouver's inner city (BC Housing 2019b). During the years before and after the Olympics, these hotels were renovated into government-subsidized supportive housing for various at-risk populations, including young people entrenched in homelessness and addiction (BC Housing 2019a; Murray 2011). This was in addition to the construction of over a dozen entirely new supportive housing sites in downtown Vancouver (City of Vancouver 2023), funded by the state and managed via partnerships between a provincial social housing agency (BC Housing), the Vancouver Coastal Health Authority (VCH), and the Ministry of Social Development and Poverty Reduction (welfare). As with privately owned SROs, rent payments for supportive housing rooms are deducted directly from monthly income assistance payments. The facilities are operated by a handful of community-based, nonprofit social housing agencies, some of which have a long history of operating in the city (Lupick 2017). Some supportive housing buildings are classified as "community care facilities" under the provincial Community Care and Assisted Living Act, which allows individuals to be released from the hospital, juvenile detention, and jail (often via the community drug court) directly into the care of these facilities (Government of BC 2020a). There, young people's traceability is facilitated by CCTV cameras and computerized fob systems, through lengthy intake questionnaires administered each time someone crosses a new institutional threshold, and by databases and files that can be accessed by various workers and teams (Boyd et al. 2016). Individual pathologies are managed via bureaucratic partnerships between various state and nonstate actors and addressed through the delivery of integrated primary, substance use, and mental health care.

The emergence of this new regime of community care was catalyzed by several events beyond the 2010 Olympics, including the downsizing and eventual closure of Riverview Psychiatric Hospital in 2012 (which at its peak held upward of five thousand patients) as part of a more general move toward deinstitutionalization in Canada (Morrow et al. 2010). Perhaps most influential to local discussions were a series of particularly damning Vancouver Police Department (VPD) reports (Thompson 2010; VPD 2009, 2013; Wilson-Bates 2008), which underscored a "surge in people with severe, untreated mental illness and addictions at St. Paul's Hospital, a dramatic increase in people taken into police custody under the Mental Health Act, and several violent episodes that indicated a major crisis in the health care system" (City of Vancouver 2014, 4). These reports framed deinstitutionalization as an epic failure in need of immediate remedy on the streets of downtown Vancouver.[2] Heavily influenced by the police reports, in 2013 the municipal government declared that Vancouver was amid a dangerous mental health crisis. A churn of meetings, task force creation, workshops, and report writing quickly ensued. Ten months later, a publication titled "Caring for All: Priority Actions to Address Mental Health and Addictions" (City of Vancouver 2014) argued for a "housing first" approach to solving the now twinned crises of mental health and addictions, "aggressively supported by appropriate community based treatment and other key supports" (8), including the police.[3] While housing first approaches are generally informed by an ethic of deinstitutionalization, the VPD and task force reports suggested a turning of the political tide back toward reinstitutionalization as a solution to the increasing visibility of homelessness, poverty, and addiction (Boyd and Kerr 2016; Morrow, Dagg, and Pederson 2008). Moreover, it was clear that the soft left hand of the state was to continue to be paired with the hard right hand of criminalization, albeit in new ways. In the past the police commonly picked up young people for loitering and shepherded them into shelters, SROs, and hospital emergency rooms. By 2013 officers viewed themselves as playing a frontline role in stabilizing at-risk youth inside these places (Bellett 2013). This shift began with the 2008 Partners in Action protocol, which assigned individual beat officers to specific supportive housing sites as a way of enhancing collaboration and information sharing between the police and housing agency staff when dealing with tenant issues, such as evictions (BC Ministry of Housing and Social Development 2008). Dealing with tenant issues also increasingly came to include apprehensions of young people under the BC Mental Health Act (BC Representative for Children and Youth 2021), which allows the police to take an individual to a physician for examination if officers believe that the person is acting in a manner likely to endanger their own safety or that of others and "is a person with a mental disorder" (Government of BC 2020b).[4] Individuals who are committed under the Mental Health Act are held for assessment in a psychiatric hospital or unit until they are deemed ready for release by a physician. If the attending psychiatrist is not confident in the patient's ability or intention to continue voluntary psychiatric treatment, they are released on "Extended Leave," oftentimes directly into the care of a supportive housing facility. There, young people must often adhere to medication regimens, which if not met lead to forcible readmission to in-patient care (Van Veen, Ibrahim, and Morrow 2018).

In 2012 VCH's Assertive Community Treatment (ACT) teams were created to further facilitate interagency collaboration and information sharing between care providers and law enforcement (VCH 2023b). While overtly aggressive and violent policing continued, it at least partially shifted toward more collaborative forms of governance characterized by enhanced surveillance and information sharing, justified by discourses of community, care, and safety (Ericson and Haggerty 1997). The inclusion of police officers in ACT teams is a made-in-Vancouver deviation from the original model that emerged during the deinstitutionalization era in North America, parts of Western Europe, Australia, and New Zealand (Killaspy et al. 2009; Phillips et al. 2001; Udechuku et al. 2005). In Vancouver ACT teams include nurses, psychiatrists, addiction counselors, social workers, peer advocates, and police officers, who work within supportive housing to provide certain residents (many on Extended Leave) with integrated primary, substance use, and mental health care—by force if necessary (Van Veen, Ibrahim, and Morrow 2018; Van Veen, Teghtsoonian, and Morrow 2019).

PATTY AND JOE, LAKESHORE HOTEL, 2010

By 2012 most of those I knew had been moved into supportive housing facilities that merged care and enforcement. But even prior to 2012 cycles of eviction and street-based homelessness began to look more like regular transfers between different supportive housing buildings run by the same social housing agency. Over time young people's biggest fear was no longer that they would find nowhere to go. Rather, they worried about getting stuck in a building that was "even worse" than the one they were leaving. For Patty and Joe in the summer of 2010, even worse referred to a building like the Lakeshore—a yet-to-be-renovated building located on a heavily gentrifying edge of the Downtown Eastside.

Earlier that same summer Patty was hospitalized for several weeks with endocarditis. At the time of her hospitalization she was facing yet another eviction from the Mackenzie Hotel for sneaking Joe into her room. Since Patty had been moved into the Mackenzie, Joe had been sleeping over almost every night, even though he still had a room at the Trafalgar Hotel. But Patty was barred from the Trafalgar, so the couple attempted to stay together at the Mackenzie. Eventually Joe was barred from the Mackenzie, leading the two of them to start sleeping outside to stay together. While spending time outside together, Patty developed endocarditis and had to be hospitalized. While she was in the hospital Patty and Joe were told by an outreach worker that they would both be moving into the Lakeshore Hotel after Patty was released.

Shortly after she and Joe moved in, one of the other residents told Patty that the Lakeshore was for the "hardest to house" people in the city; it was the "end of the line" in terms of where they could put "people like her and Joe." Everyone knew that the Lakeshore was one of "the worst" buildings in downtown Vancouver. Yet it was located in the middle of one of the trendiest and most expensive neighborhoods in the city, where the historic stone and brick warehouses, hotels, and storefronts that grew up around the prosperity of the Canadian Pacific Railway at the turn of the twentieth century had been carefully restored into office spaces, restaurants, and boutiques. People with money from all over Greater Vancouver and the world flocked to Patty and Joe's neighborhood to enjoy its amenities and ambiance, for some made even more alluring by its proximity to the Downtown Eastside. As a prominent luxury condo development in the neighborhood advertised in 2006, wealthy frequenters of

Patty and Joe's neighborhood were challenged to either "be bold or move to suburbia."

Patty and Joe lived at the Lakeshore for two years. During that time I visited with them regularly in the cramped and chronically untidy room that they shared. Although they had been allotted separate rooms, they lived in one room and used the other for storage and for "time-outs" when they were having a particularly bad fight. They were able to let in some fresh air through a single, curtain-less window, but it did little to reduce the smell of stale cigarette smoke and mildewed clothing. Particularly during the cold and wet winter months, it was difficult to dry out clothing and shoes made permanently damp by the rain. During the summer months their room became stiflingly hot, and large clouds of insects ascended in flight any time their bare double mattress or piles of belongings were disturbed. Prior to renovation the Lakeshore continued to be infested with insects and rodents. Sinks and toilets clogged up and overflowed. Our conversations there were regularly interrupted by yelling in the hallway and pounding on doors. Some of the antics in the hallway were humorous, others were menacing.

Patty and Joe seemed to spend much of their time at the Lakeshore dreaming of living somewhere else. During this period Patty started talking more frequently about wanting to go home to Edmonton for a while to reconnect with her family and take a break from using drugs. Patty wanted Joe to do the same, but he was more ambivalent about returning to Saskatoon where his stepmom was living or the Northwest Territories where his dad lived. They both talked a lot about getting an apartment in the West End of downtown Vancouver, close to the colorful gay bars and nightclubs of Davie Village, or a basement suite in East Vancouver, near a cluster of Vancouver Native Housing Society buildings. Patty longed to live in an area of the city that was, as she put it, more "diverse": a neighborhood where other Indigenous people lived in "regular" housing and could be seen going about their daily lives in the absence of the everyday emergencies of unstable housing and homelessness, and where she could feel comfortable going into shops to buy food, browse used clothing, and try on makeup without worrying whether someone was going to call the cops on her. In their current neighborhood Patty and Joe *were* the diversity that a daily influx of working professionals, restaurant patrons, and tourists simultaneously feared and desired: they were brown skinned and visibly poor and addicted to drugs. Patty and Joe longed instead to live amid the kind of diversity that would make them less visible: in a neighborhood where they could blend in as just another young couple trying to figure their lives out, coming and going from their place of residence to shop, relax together, hang out with friends, and perhaps eventually work or go back to school.

LOSING EVERYTHING

Evictions and building transfers were often followed up with drug and alcohol relapses, binges, and mental health crises. In the chaos of each move, young people often angrily described losing everything. This sense of loss referred to material possessions; in the wake of the conflicts and crises that almost always surrounded these moves they would simply abandon their possessions or were forced to abandon them because of periods of hospitalization or incarceration. But the sense of loss they experienced went beyond their things. Over time, frequent moves had the effect of dislocating them from place, and from each other.[5] The forms of sociality once embedded in places like the Lighthouse shelter and the Mackenzie and Trafalgar hotels were significantly eroded as they were transferred from building to building and spent time in the hospital and jail. Across time and place, young people noticed that they were somehow moving further away from their dreams of place in the city rather than toward them. They began to describe themselves as lost in the city.

PATTY AND JOE, ST. MARY'S, 2012

In the winter of 2012 Patty and Joe were abruptly moved out of the Lakeshore because it was finally scheduled for renovation. They were transferred into a recently renovated supportive housing building in the Downtown South that included a dedicated floor and program (YouthNow) for young people with mental health and addiction issues. St. Mary's was located only a few blocks away from both the old Lighthouse shelter and the Trafalgar and MacKenzie hotels.

Over the previous two years Patty and Joe had complained frequently about living at the Lakeshore Hotel. However, when they were told to pack up their stuff (and were paid five hundred dollars each for their cooperation), Patty suddenly began reflecting on the fragile sense of family that she and Joe had managed to create there. "When you lose something, that's when you realize what you really had," Patty remarked sadly on the day they moved out. Rain plastered her hair to her face as she loaded several sagging garbage bags of stuff into a housing agency van. "Now we really feel homeless. Again." Patty and so many others continued to use the language of homelessness to describe their circumstances, even though they were increasingly transferred directly from one building to another.

Entering St. Mary's in 2012, it was not hard to understand why young people consistently described a rupture between "the old days" of chaotic shelters and rundown buildings like the Lighthouse, the Trafalgar, and the Mackenzie—in which they nevertheless "ran things"—and "the new days" of supportive housing.[6] The interior of St. Mary's was bathed in neon light. The vintage black-and-white tile floors might actually have been charming if it wasn't for the monochrome white paint job that glowed a yellowish green under the harsh fluorescent lighting. The hotel entrance, once a rowdy meeting spot, had become a site of surveillance, with closed-circuit security cameras and a glassed-in reception desk with multiple computer screens. The effect was such that several supportive housing buildings have been used as sets for law-and-order television shows—including as the interior of a police station (Boyd et al. 2016). A computerized fob system limited access to other floors, so that residents and guests were no longer permitted to move freely throughout the building and between rooms. Front desk sign-in procedures that required leaving a government-issued ID discouraged frequent visitors and also meant that those who were able to enter—often relying on a sympathetic staff person willing to overlook the ID requirement—would commonly spend inordinate amounts of time in a single room out of fear that if they left they would be unable to get back in. On some building floors, glass-paned offices and medical rooms backed onto common areas that now largely remained empty. In contrast to the lively, turbulent atmosphere at the Lighthouse, the Trafalgar, and the Mackenzie, at St. Mary's young people described themselves as "sitting around all day" in their individual rooms, listening for the footsteps and jingling keys of staff as they made half-hourly inspections.[7]

"It's desolate," was how Joe described it, shortly after he and Patty had moved in. The three of us were sitting together in the small room they shared. Patty and Joe both looked tired, their eyes ringed with dark circles. During those first months at St. Mary's, they told me that they found it impossible to sleep. Instead, they used meth to stay awake outside through the night. Sometimes Joe wandered off on his own, lost in reveries and hallucinations that were unknowable to anyone but him. He had done this for as long as Patty had known him, but since moving into St. Mary's it had been happening more often.

Joe continued, "It feels like the walls are caving in on your head. Impending doom. Nobody's around, anymore. They separated us all from each other. Patty and me are on our own here."

"It's just like jail, basically," Patty sighed. "Especially juvie [juvenile detention]. Jingle, jingle, jingle. I hate it."

The room that Patty and Joe moved into had been freshly painted. It was clean and free of insects and rodents. But Patty said that the austere white walls reminded her of "institutions." Many young people compared supportive housing rooms to jail cells and hospital wards, describing how each of these places evoked similar senses of containment ("it feels like the walls are caving in on your head"), isolation ("nobody's around"), and surveillance.

A sense of entrapment may seem at odds with a sense of getting lost, which implies not knowing one's whereabouts. And yet young people frequently articulated senses of both getting trapped and getting lost as they attempted to understand where they had ended up in the city. When they used the language of getting lost in the context of their supportive housing buildings—and to describe their sense of place in Vancouver more generally—they seemed to be evoking the multiple meanings of the word lost: a sense of not knowing (or perhaps not understanding) one's whereabouts and a sense of something that has been taken away. Getting lost seemed to refer to the feeling that they were somehow moving further away from the lives they wanted for themselves. They were increasingly "fixed in place" (Roe 2009/2010, 75) and "fixed in time" (Murray 2015, 293), unable to actualize desired futures.

A sense of getting lost was also tied to various kinds of disappearance. As described earlier, there were many ways individuals could disappear from the city for periods of time, including drug binges that kept them indoors somewhere, or moving quickly from place to place, for days on end. They frequently had to lie low and hide or keep moving. They were hospitalized and went to jail, detox, and treatment. There were also more permanent forms of disappearance, including death.

Patty and Joe acknowledged that supportive housing buildings were much safer than the old shelters and SROs, yet these forms of disappearance persisted, even intensified. "Since we've been moved out of the Lakeshore, three of our friends—or ex-neighbors—have died," Patty reflected. During this time, their own drug use had escalated. After two and a half years clean off heroin, Patty had begun using it again and was regularly "falling off" (discontinuing) her methadone. Joe was also using meth and heroin and was on and off methadone. Patty had started talking again about how she and Joe needed to leave the city and return home to visit family for a time.

"It's so much more dangerous here than we thought when we first came to Vancouver. There might not be as many murders here as in Edmonton [due to gang violence in this Canadian city], but there's a lot of"—Patty searched for the word—"statistics? Here. Anybody can do drugs in these rooms and not have the door open and they could just overdose. You know, like, the [harm reduction] supplies are all there, it's so easy to use—and two days later they could find your body. Or you could die in hospital, and nobody would ever hear from you again. Or just—" she trailed off. "Yeah. We keep losing people. This one guy, he-he died just recently. He was a meth dealer, and they-they found him in his new room with ten thousand dollars under his mattress. He overdosed, we think. It was like, as soon as they got, like, moved out of the Lakeshore, they all, like, had mental breakdowns, or—"

"Like, you might get your fifteen minutes of-of fame [in the drug-dealing game] here," Joe interrupted. He added softly, "But then, we can get lost after. You could die. Someone else takes your spot [dealing drugs]. Overdose. Go crazy. These places [supportive housing buildings] are a dead end."

"I miss how it used to be, back when it was more social, and, like, everyone knew everyone and we were all together," Patty said nostalgically. "We didn't have to live inside these buildings and be all isolated and get all sketchy and paranoid because you're doing drugs on your own in your room all the time. It's kinda horrible, now. It's not a good feeling."

BOREDOM

A sense of getting lost in supportive housing could also be closely aligned with experiences of boredom. While previous work on boredom and modernity asserts that boredom is a problem of excess—of having a lot of nothing (Goodstein 2005)—anthropologists working in settings of entrenched poverty have noted that locating boredom in the capitalist dichotomization of work and leisure time does not account for what free time means in such contexts. For those I knew, as elsewhere, unstructured time could become an overabundant and even dangerous quantity (Mains 2012), and boredom seemed to derive from being both over- and *under*whelmed (Jervis, Spicer, and Manson 2003; Masquelier 2019; Musharbash 2007; O'Neill 2014). A crushing sense of boredom inside supportive housing could be a powerful register of distress related to the experience of reaching a kind of dead end in terms of the ability to actualize a future different from the past and present (Mains 2012; O'Neill 2014). The chronology of youth—a category powerfully embedded with notions of progress—shaped the devastation of chronic boredom for many. Across time, boredom could engender the feeling that, instead of achieving some kind of upward—or at least forward—mobility, young people were somehow drifting further and further away from their dreams of place.

AARON, NORTHWEST APARTMENTS, 2013

Within supportive housing, various aspects of daily life are unified. In contrast to the old days of SROs and shelters when young people often had to do their own harm reduction from their backpacks, clean needles and other drug use paraphernalia are all readily available inside buildings, handed out by building staff and managers. In these places a diffused mode of governmentality flows through the bloodstream in the form of opioid agonist therapies like methadone and buprenorphine-naloxone (brand name Suboxone) and psychopharmacotherapies like risperidone, quetiapine, olanzapine, and aripiprazole (brand name Abilify), which can be delivered right to young people's doors by members of the ACT teams and other outreach workers. Buildings are visited regularly by other professionals as well, including social workers and probation officers. There are daily hot meal programs and free coffee. A range of social services—from a weekly photography club to a comprehensive, youth-focused mental health and addiction program (YouthNow)—are run right out of some buildings.

Young people's experiences of these different forms of care varied. Often within the very same conversation they might angrily describe getting absolutely no help at all from building staff and outreach workers and then tell a moving story about how these same individuals had saved their lives. Most had at least one outreach worker in their lives for whom they genuinely cared and who they felt cared for them. When they aged out of these relationships at age nineteen and then again at around twenty-five, they were devastated.

At the same time, most of those I knew were less concerned with the positives and negatives of particular kinds of supportive housing programming than with the general fact that these places seemed to constitute a form of (re)institutionalization—one that had occurred without their explicit consent or at the very least full knowledge of "what the hell was going on," as Aaron put it in 2013. These were places where young people's moves were increasingly traced and decided by others. Many entered supportive housing buildings via court mandates and Extended Leave agreements; failure to comply with these living arrangements could mean hospitalization or jail time. Court-mandated living arrangements were often accompanied by red zones and probation conditions that further limited their movements: they had to stay not only in the city but often in the immediate vicinity of their supportive housing building. The forms of care embedded in supportive housing could map seamlessly onto these forms of control. They were also a means of encouraging young people to stay put: these were the places where they were now expected to eat their meals and drink their coffee and access medications and harm reduction supplies. This was where a significant portion of their welfare checks went each month and where they could access contingency management programs that included a weekly gift certificate draw (an additional source of income for some).[8] All these measures were intended to help young people. Yet the effect for some was a sense that supportive housing was simply one more in a long line of institutions to be endured.

Since 2009 Aaron had cycled through five different buildings operated by the same social housing agency—he had been through all of them. In 2013, he was evicted from St. Mary's over an altercation with staff and transferred into another facility that he was assured would be "a step up" in terms of finally finding a permanent place to live. The fact that the facility was called Northwest Apartments was particularly misleading—Aaron assumed, initially, that he was being moved into what he thought of as a "real" apartment building. Instead, he found himself in what he described as a low security hospital.

Sitting in the field office in the Downtown South in the fall of 2013, Aaron reflected angrily, "St. Mary's, the YouthNow program, Northwest Apartments—they're basically trying to manage my life again, and set up appointments and make decisions for me when I'm not aware of it—like, trying to get me to take meds." He and Laurie had shown up soaked from the rain, each weighed down by a large backpack and carrying additional garbage bags full of stuff that altogether outsized their small frames. Upon arriving, they both piled their things in a corner and peeled off their outer layers of wet clothes, hanging them to dry over the row of chairs in the lobby. Laurie prepared them both coffees with milk and an ample amount of sugar and then set to work on making peanut butter and jam sandwiches. Aaron was halfway through his second one as he explained, "You can only be in that [YouthNow] program and get all the help and shit they give you—like help with getting your ID and groceries, and [field]trips and pizza lunches and gift cards and *all* that stuff—if you agree to go see a doctor, right? They *make* you see a doctor. And then he tries to get you to take meds and shit. He wanted me to take Seroquel. And he asked me to go be a guinea pig for medications. You get paid twenty bucks, but they make you sign this sheet that says any side effects or anything—you can't sue them and shit. I know some people that are messed up now, that are in that YouthNow program. Well, they were f-cked up before, but now they are a different kind of messed up. They're zombies, man."

I had noticed the same thing as Aaron. It seemed to me that, since moving into supportive housing, a much larger proportion of those I knew—in particular young men—were on antipsychotic medications, including those delivered in the form of a monthly injection.[9] These once loud and unruly individuals had become quieter and more subdued, and I had often wondered if that was a good thing.

Brushing the crumbs from his standard, monochrome uniform of a black hoody and track suit pants, Aaron said, "In the place I'm in now, they've got a *meds room.* Actually *in* the building. All of the people living there are mentally ill."

I asked Aaron bluntly, "Do you consider yourself mentally ill?"

"I'm not mentally ill," he replied matter-of-factly. "That's why I quit the Youth-Now program. That's why I'm getting out of there."

Aaron was soon transferred to yet another supportive housing facility, this time run by a different social housing agency, after another altercation with staff. He later told me that when he got kicked out of Northwest Apartments they used the word "discharged" rather than "evicted."

The experience of being (re)institutionalized in supportive housing could be powerfully racialized and bound up with previous experiences of being moved between government foster care and group homes, juvenile detention and correctional centers, and hospitals.[10] Aaron is Kwanlin Dün First Nations. He grew up in Whitehorse (a city in a northern Canadian territory), entering government care when he was one and a half years old and spending many of his childhood years in the same group home. There, he developed a close relationship with a social worker, who "stayed with him" throughout his childhood. Eventually, at age eight he was moved into a receiving home in anticipation of being adopted into a family. He stayed there, waiting, for a long time. Finally, he was told that he would not be adopted after all. He was moved back into his first group home and then eventually into another group home for teenagers at age thirteen. When he was a child, Aaron recalled regularly imagining what it might be like to be adopted into a family. However, as he was moved across different homes and the possibility of adoption became increasingly remote, he told me that he "trained his mind" not to focus on the future.

By the time Aaron was in his midteens he was cycling through social worker after social worker and running away regularly from his group home to spend time with his aunties, uncles, and cousins. He had not known these family members as a child but was able to get to know them during adolescence. He started getting arrested on various charges and spending time in the White-horse RCMP's "drunk tank," Yukon Young Offenders Facility, and, eventually, the Whitehorse Correctional Centre. He told me that when he was seventeen he was tricked into going to a rehabilitation center in Alberta for "out of control Native kids." On the day that he was escorted by police to the Whitehorse Airport to board a plane to Edmonton, he was told by group home staff that they needed to have a meeting with him at his school about his lack of attendance. He later learned that they had lied; the plan had been to take him to the airport all along. Aaron skipped school that day and missed the meeting but was picked up on the street by a police officer who had previously taken him snowboarding as part of a local youth program. The group home van pulled up alongside them, and Aaron was forced inside. He was flown to Edmonton with only the clothes he was wearing. From then on, at the rehabilitation center in Alberta and at the group home once he returned to Whitehorse, Aaron's plan was to "take care of things on his own." He ran away consistently to spend time on the streets and with his family, until, when he turned nineteen, he made his way down to Vancouver, using money he received when he aged out of govern-ment care.

Aaron was haunted by the violence he experienced in his second group home and in the rehabilitation center. In both places, after running away and being tracked down, he was physically roughed up and locked in his room for what felt to him like weeks, the windows boarded up so that he could not leave. Supportive housing buildings were not the same as these places, of course: young people could leave if they wanted to. So why did Aaron and many others regularly compare supportive housing to locked-down institutional settings such as rehabilitation, juvenile detention and correctional centers, and psychiatric wards?

For Aaron, supportive housing environments echoed previous moments in his life, when he had been promised something that was then yanked away (then: adoption into a family, now: a normal apartment) and when he was tricked into doing something he didn't want or think he needed (then: attending a rehabilitation program for "out of control Native kids," now: living in a building for "mentally ill" people and being strongly pressured to take psychiatric medications). Aaron told me once that as a child he only ever knew "shift change," only knew social workers and other professionals coming and going, their plans for his life coming and going just as quickly. In and across supportive housing environments, shift change continued: building managers, staff, and outreach workers cycled through and moved on, and young people aged out of particular programs and services, abruptly finding themselves without access to those professionals with whom they had developed relationships.

"It's all the same—it's all more of the same," Aaron said to me in 2014. I had asked him about what kind of future he imagined for himself in the city. We were sitting in the field office again because Aaron never invited me to visit him in or around the places where he lived. He seemed to like coming to our field office, though, which he said was the only "service" he regularly accessed. He would hang around anywhere from twenty minutes to several hours, making himself coffee and food, using the phone, watching TV, and picking through our donated clothing and toiletries for anything he might need or be able to sell.

"I don't think about that kind of stuff," he continued, sighing heavily and shifting on his chair suddenly, seeming to indicate that he was going to get up and leave. My question had irritated him in a way that seemed to simultaneously create a sense of fatigue. It was a reaction I had seen many times among those I followed, usually in response to well-meaning encouragement from providers, workers, and professionals to engage in some kind of planning or goal setting. Many young people seemed to like spending time with me imagining what their futures might look like: the kinds of places they might live in, the jobs they might have, the relationships with romantic partners and children and pets that they might nurture, the leisure activities with which they might eventually fill their time. Others, like Aaron, were not interested in doing this—with me, at least. Across time and geographies, a sense of being perpetually out of place seemed to powerfully shape not only how the present was perceived and acted upon but also whether it was preferable to imagine a future at all.

(NO)EXIT, SHAE, 2013

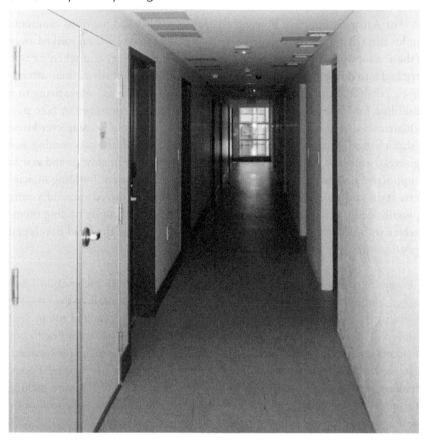

FLASHBACKS AND FUTURES

While life at St. Mary's was a stark contrast to that at the Lighthouse, the Mackenzie, and the Trafalgar, it had significant continuity with young people's experiences of institutionalization. Glassed-in reception desks, CCTV cameras, fob systems, and locked-off floors could resurface distressing memories and flashbacks of time spent in hospital and psychiatric wards, juvenile detention centers, and jail.[11]

The mechanisms of surveillance and control built into supportive housing are intended to increase the safety of residents and staff. Places like St. Mary's and Northwest Apartments were safer than the old Trafalgar and Mackenzie hotels in terms of the risk of physical and sexual violence. Unlike in the old buildings, in supportive housing facilities it was possible to securely lock the door to your room and keep unwanted individuals out. Building managers and staff constantly kept an eye on things. On several occasions I saw them kick out or bar men who were attempting to crash in young women's rooms for indefinite periods, with the intention of sharing the money and drugs largely procured through the latter's sex work.

Yet despite the various safety measures in place, supportive housing environments could simultaneously signal a pressing sense of danger. Those I knew had survived by paying attention to these kinds of signals across their young lives and knowing when to get out, to get away. A finely tuned sense of danger could be powerfully racialized. For Indigenous young people, it was cultivated through experiences of institutionalization that extended across their own lives and generations. Faced with this sense of danger, many fled their supportive housing buildings for as long as they possibly could without facing another building transfer. They used crystal meth to stay awake and outside for long stretches of time. Others stayed inside their buildings, using increasing amounts of drugs to dull the sense that something was terribly wrong.

The disjuncture between life in supportive housing and the futures that young people imagined in the city could also fuel escalating levels of drug use.[12] As they were moved into these buildings, most remained deeply invested in alternative dreams of place. Somewhat paradoxically, these dreams could include living in the gentrifying neighborhoods where St. Mary's and the Lakeshore Hotel were located. Once there, however, they contended with a growing sense of dispossession (Garcia 2010) from what was all around them yet increasingly out of reach. Mostly, they vehemently rejected the notion that supportive housing constituted a "real home." What was at stake was not just that supportive housing did not feel permanent, given frequent evictions and building transfers, but also that these places *could not* feel permanent because this would mean that young people belonged there—in places that were for the mentally ill and addicted.

PATTY, TERMINAL CITY, 2013

"The heroin's been getting really good lately," Patty remarked at the beginning of 2013. The Terminal City was perpetually shades of gray, the rain relentless.[13] "It's gotten a lot stronger lately. And it's everywhere," she laughed nervously. "There's a lot more of it around, suddenly."

THE DANCE OF DEATH

The escalation of drug use among some young people within supportive housing highlights an alarming contradiction.[14] These facilities are tasked with the protection of life through the increased surveillance and regulation of the human body. However, sitting alone in their rooms, getting higher than ever by fine-tuning combinations of illicit drugs and licit pharmaceuticals, young people increasingly acknowledged that they lived with the possibility of overdose and death. For some, there was a troubling sense that the dance of death in which they were embroiled was orchestrated by the state, which provided the housing, welfare money, and harm reduction supplies. By 2012 these supplies included take-home naloxone (brand name Narcan) overdose antidote kits, which were becoming increasingly necessary to resuscitate people who had "gone down."

As they found themselves withdrawing into more and more solitary practices inside supportive housing, many young people also found themselves progressively more wired to what they thought was heroin. Some reflected on a kind of symmetry between their shifting drug use and the places where they lived. The hyperstimulating effects of meth seemed to mirror the frenetic, communal atmosphere of places like the Lighthouse shelter and Mackenzie and Trafalgar hotels, while the languorous, inward-turning effects of opioids reflected the more isolating worlds of buildings like St. Mary's. An opioid addiction seemed to make more sense to some in terms of where they were currently living; it mellowed them out, made them less social, and allowed them to sleep for long periods. But a cruel coincidence was also at play. Concerted efforts to move young people into supportive housing coincided with the arrival of illicitly manufactured fentanyl in Vancouver sometime during 2011 (Lupick 2017). The introduction into the local drug supply of synthetic fentanyl, ten times stronger than heroin, caused the number of fatal overdoses to jump by nearly a third (from 211 to 295) that year alone. Yet even in 2013 none of those I knew had any clear idea that this was why the heroin had "gotten really good" and was "a lot stronger" and "everywhere"—or why people seemed to be overdosing all around them. It would be three more years before an overdose public health emergency was declared, and many of those whom I was close to began to die.

PATTY AND JOE, ST. MARY'S, 2013

I visited Patty and Joe in the various rooms that they lived in over the years. More often, however, they suggested that we spend time together elsewhere, at fast-food restaurants, public parks, and beaches. I was therefore surprised one day when Patty told me that she wanted to show me her recently tidied room at St. Mary's. Welcoming me in with a ceremonious "ta-da!," she and Joe settled themselves on a single bed carefully made up with a shiny synthetic emerald green comforter and two small, yellowed pillows. The late afternoon sun filtered through the window, lighting the sides of their faces. I sat opposite them on a hard laminate and metal chair, lodged between a metal sink area and an older model television still covered in its plastic casing and balanced precariously atop a small table. In every corner of the room there were piles of neatly tied plastic shopping bags filled with clothing and other possessions. A small painting of a tropical beach was propped up in the window. Despite how often young people talked about hating the places where they were living, I regularly observed the many ways in which they attempted to transform their rooms and camps into homes.

It was spring 2013. Patty's optimism that day was shaped by a promise made to her and Joe back in 2012, when they had left the Lakeshore Hotel and moved into St. Mary's. At that time they were told by a housing agency manager that former residents of the Lakeshore would be given "first dibs" on the renovated rooms there. And, as a couple, Patty and Joe would be eligible for one of the few larger suites in the building, with self-contained kitchenettes and their own bathrooms. During the months that followed, Patty and Joe regularly expressed their excitement at the possibility of moving into what they envisioned would be a normal, two-person apartment. They diligently followed up with the housing agency over and over again, trying to confirm with a rotation of managers that they would ultimately hold up their end of the bargain. Finally, on that day in her tidied room, Patty happily informed me that one housing agency manager had finally followed up with her about moving back into the Lakeshore after the renovations were complete.

In the meantime, at St. Mary's, Patty and Joe endeavored to spend as little time there as possible. Even through the cold winter months of 2013, they spent much of their time outside, where rushed hits of meth and heroin took place in filthy back alleys and parking lots. Patty worried that she might develop another infection and have to be hospitalized again. Instead, it was Joe who had to be hospitalized for two months in early 2014, when he contracted endocarditis.

Patty and Joe continued to debate going home or to treatment to escape St. Mary's. From Patty's perspective, this became more urgent when Joe was hospitalized. During those rare times when she left Joe's bedside, Patty found a long-term residential treatment and recovery program in a suburb of Greater Vancouver that appealed to her because it allowed couples to attend together. Patty and Joe had no intention of separating to attend residential treatment programs. Like every other couple I knew, they vowed to stay together no matter what and insisted that was the only way they would ever be able to address their substance use and mental health issues. However, when Patty mentioned her and Joe's plan to attend a treatment program for couples to a housing agency staff member, she was told that leaving their rooms at St. Mary's for an indefinite period would mean not only losing their rooms there but also forfeiting the possibility of securing one of the larger apartments in the Lakeshore. In the end, when Joe was released on Extended Leave from the hospital, he and Patty were "sent straight back" to St. Mary's.

Sitting with me at a nearby park a few days later, Patty reflected despondently, "We're like, trying to get out of the system, and they just push you back in. It's confusing because, like, we wanna go to treatment but we also don't wanna lose a good place [at the renovated Lakeshore Hotel]. I mean, what if treatment didn't work out?"

She sighed. "Ultimately, we do have the choice to leave, but it doesn't really feel like we have the choice to leave. We don't belong there [at St. Mary's]. We're just kind of lost down here at this point—with what to do at this point. I don't want to be one of those girls, you know, stuck down here—like, they're skinny, they've got that hunchback from the down [opioids]. They're hopeless. They're never going to *not* be that way. I don't want to end up like that. Because what kind of life is that? That's not what I want for our future."

WHERE WE'VE ENDED UP, PATTY AND JOE, 2013

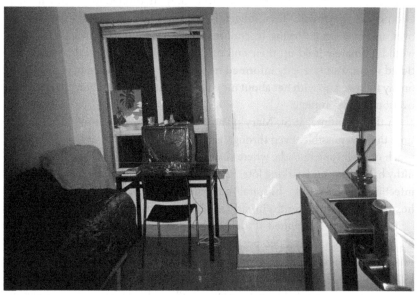

WAITING

Those I knew were deeply engaged in trying to make homes and families and lives for themselves in Vancouver. Sitting around in supportive housing and the various elsewheres to which they routinely escaped, they struggled to reconcile particular dreams of place with where they had ended up. In certain moments utopian imaginaries of home allowed them to reconfigure their senses of place and self in the city. In other moments they expressed the need to be realistic about the kinds of homes they would ultimately be able to make in the city. They diligently filled out paperwork and made the calls (and follow-up calls) to ensure that they were on the waiting list for better social housing, such as a two-person self-contained apartment in a renovated supportive housing building or a government-subsidized condominium in prime developments like the Olympic Village or Woodward's complexes. Almost everyone I knew believed that they were on a BC Housing waiting list for one of the latter—a list that was rumored to be so long it took seven years to get a place.

But for some being realistic seemed to mean not thinking about the future at all. Often expediated by the intensive use of drugs and alcohol, this was a powerful antidote to the agony of waiting for your life to change.

TERRY, ST. MARY'S, 2014

While many felt unmoored by their moves into and across supportive housing sites, others could be held up as examples of how these places had the potential to stabilize even the most "severely drug addicted, mentally ill, [and] hard to house" young people—a characterization that was carried around by most of those I knew (Wilson-Bates 2008, 38). During the six years I had known him Terry had cycled in and out of numerous shelters and SROs and countless periods of homelessness and incarceration. Upon getting out of jail for yet another shoplifting-related charge in 2012, however, Terry was released into the care of an emergency shelter in the Downtown Eastside and then transferred to St. Mary's. He lived on the same youth-dedicated floor that Patty, Joe, Aaron, and Laurie had all passed through and was (briefly) enrolled in the YouthNow program.

Whereas once it had been almost impossible for me to remain in regular contact with Terry, over the following two years I was able to visit him regularly. Each time I entered St. Mary's I offered my government ID to the person at the glassed-in reception desk but was frequently told that it wasn't required from service providers (although I never identified myself that way). I took the stairs to Terry's floor, which included another glassed-in office, laundry facilities, and common area with a laminated calendar tacked up on the wall, indicating when various YouthNow group activities took place.

Sitting together in his meticulously tidied room in the early summer of 2014, Terry was positive and optimistic. He began our conversation that day by telling me how much he loved it at St. Mary's—his room, the staff, the free coffee—and how happy he was to have what he referred to, rather opaquely at first, as a daily routine. Each day he woke up and took the bus to a popular drop-in center in the Downtown Eastside to have breakfast, before returning by bus to the Downtown South to begin his "work day."

As we talked, I studied the various items carefully placed on a single shelf across from his bed, above a long metal counter with sink. Framed photographs of his brother and sister and a weathered scrapbook of newspaper clippings were propped up ceremoniously amid several candles and an iPod dock. I asked if I could look through the scrapbook (which Terry then told me was put together by his grandma) and saw that all of the stories were feel-good pieces about animals: a baby crocodile found in someone's basement, a cat that wears clothing. Terry then encouraged me to look through a plastic file folder that was sitting on the counter and contained the numerous documents he needed for various appointments. Plastic labels with the words "welfare" and "disability" peeked out from between heavily crumpled sheets of paper, which I glanced at only quickly. The postcard I had sent him from one of my trips to Tanzania was tacked up on the wall, beside a long list of Sharpied phone numbers—his drug-dealing connections, he told me.

Eventually that day Terry was more explicit about how stable housing had allowed him to move beyond risky, grab-and-run shoplifting as his primary means of income generation. In 2014 Terry's routine involved selling hash and unregulated cigarettes up and down Granville Street. During the years he lived there, the walls of his room at St. Mary's were at times covered with inspirational graffiti and writing similar to that which appeared in the diaries and letters he had written for me while in jail. Much of it was meant to remind him of his target income for the day (e.g., "$100 → $200"). By this time Terry had been kicked out of the YouthNow program for failing to follow through on the kinds of goal set-ting that were a part of the contingency management therapy they offered. Even-tually he was also too old to be eligible for the program. Once he was no longer allowed to participate in YouthNow's weekly gift certificate draw, he had begun collecting these gift certificates from others still in the program and procuring drugs for them in return. In return for facilitating this transaction, Terry took a share of the procured opioids and meth. For a time he was also using an HP Photosmart printer to produce counterfeit twenty-dollar bills in his room. Some mornings he told me he actually managed to use these to buy Tim Hortons cof-fee and donuts, pocketing the change.

Terry powerfully echoed others' concerns regarding the coercive nature of mental health and addiction treatment in supportive housing buildings. At one point he reflected, "I don't think I need antipsychotics, but I take them reli-giously. Most of the people that I've come across here [at St. Mary's], that are on disability welfare—about 95 percent of them—receive an injection [of anti-psychotic medication].[15] And everybody that gets injections tells me, I hate this thing. Well, I wish I could stay on my nine-hundred-dollar disability [welfare] per month without my injection! But you can't do it, right? Well, you can, but they [the ACT team] will hunt you down here and try and stick you with a needle."

However, for Terry, St. Mary's did not seem to evoke the same kinds of flash-backs or anxieties about the future as it did for many others. He did not view St. Mary's as an institution or a dead end. Instead, it was a place that opened up different kinds of possibilities—of establishing a daily routine and generating a steadier income, for example. His life there still did not look the way that various professionals might have liked. Nevertheless, it did stabilize him for some years. During his time at St. Mary's Terry largely stayed out of the hospital and jail. Eventually, after successfully selling drugs and cigarettes on Granville Street, he also occasionally began going to a local temporary work agency and picking up odd construction jobs during the morning hours, before binging on drugs in the afternoon.

FLIGHTS

Within supportive housing, young people enacted various inventions, escapes, and flights. While it had increasingly disastrous and deadly outcomes, their drug use continued to be a form of vital experimentation that opened up new social, economic, spatial, and affective possibilities in circumstances marked by stagnation, boredom, loss, flashbacks, and anxieties about the future. The achievements and defeats of dealing, debts, and crime also continued to propel them forward. Most young people's rooms were packed with stolen and collected merchandise, which they sold and traded daily. Dealing inside supportive housing was more clandestine than at the old shelters and hotels, but it was still standard practice. If they were not dealing themselves, they often bought their drugs from a dealer on the same floor as where they lived or from someone in another, nearby building. The rooms of resident dealers were sites of relative abundance and decadence in the midst of deprivation: they could be lavishly decorated with a mix of bought and traded treasures, with expensive sound systems that blared trap rap into otherwise austere hallways. These displays of wealth continually accumulated and dissolved back into circulation as individuals rose to and fell from power in the street-level drug-dealing game.

As already described, many fled their supportive housing buildings altogether. They stayed outside, moving around the city. They spent inordinate amounts of time in the privately owned SROs that still existed, where the doors to rooms remained open and it was still possible to move from floor to floor, visiting and buying and selling drugs. These places continued to be filthy and unsafe, but they were also social and communal. Some eventually decided not to go back to their buildings. While young, homeless bodies were increasingly absent from the sidewalks of the downtown core, many continued to find outdoor places to sleep in and around the fringes of Greater Vancouver.[16]

PATTY AND JOE, LAKESHORE HOTEL, 2014

In summer 2014, Patty and Joe finally got their wish: they were moved into one of the new, larger apartments at the renovated Lakeshore Hotel. When I met them at a McDonald's restaurant a few weeks before the move, Patty was positive and energized, talking a mile a minute about her decorating plans, which included the creation of a study area with two desks—one for her, one for Joe. We sat outside on the curb of a parking lot in the bright sun, burgers and fries spread out like a picnic on the warm asphalt. Joe had a slight smile on his face as he allowed Patty to do all of the talking.

"Once we're settled in and everything, we wanna continue, like, school," Patty said loudly, so that she could be heard over the sound of nearby traffic. "That's our goal—we're gonna try to get our high school. Because I only have my grade 9, and Joe has even less. We're gonna get a big room with our own bathroom and our own living room and stuff like that—and we're going to be legally common law. I can't wait, it's going to be so much better!" she gushed. "And even my grandma and my family, they're really proud of me, for getting this place and everything."

I visited Patty and Joe at their new room in the Lakeshore in the early fall of 2014, bringing with me a box of housewarming gifts that included a heart-shaped door mat, dish towels, and an intricately detailed but fake potted plant. The leaves of the trees outside their building had changed color but not yet started to fall. In certain ways their new room was what we had all imagined many times during the previous two years: u-shaped, with two decent-sized living areas (each larger than their old room at St. Mary's) connected by a kitchenette and bathroom. And yet I could tell immediately on the day of my first visit that Patty and Joe were preoccupied and unhappy. I had to awkwardly set the box of gifts on top of the kitchen counter, where it sat untouched until I was about to leave, and Patty made a last-minute effort to look through the items and thank me. She and Joe did gratefully accept the takeout coffees I had managed to carry up the stairs along with the box of gifts, and for a time we sat together in silence at a small kitchen table and chairs that looked like they had come with the room. Patty and Joe drank their coffees quickly, hungrily. I wondered if they had gone out to eat yet that day, although it was nearly two o'clock in the afternoon. As I sipped my own coffee I tried to tell which side of the unit they were using for sleeping and which side they were using for the living room and desk area that Patty had described to me the last time we saw each other. In one room I spotted a mattress on the floor, covered with stuff. In the other room there was more stuff everywhere, but no couch or desks.

"How's it going here?" I finally asked, tentatively.

Patty half-heartedly launched into what had been happening since they moved back into the building. She sounded tired. "It feels almost like a war in the building," she said. "It's full of new people, there's a new manager, and um, she-she wants to change the whole building, and she's, like, trying to evict all the old tenants [who lived at the Lakeshore pre-renovation]. She's been trying to evict me and Joe. Well, she-she actually did evict Joe, and she evicted one of my best friends for like, using [drugs] with her door open, and using in the hall. But the thing is, that's what we all know from the way it used to be at the Lakeshore. We all used—we looked at it as harm reduction, because we don't want to, like, die in our rooms with the doors closed, alone, or whatever. But now the manager and a lot of the new residents are looking at us like 'Whoa—they're, like, hard-core junkies.'"

Joe added more quietly, almost in a whisper, "She [the manager] wants to, like, separate us." He had said nothing up until that point. His thin frame was slumped down on the chair, and he was shivering despite the warmth of the room.

Acknowledging his interjection, Patty added forcefully, "If they split us up— it's not going to—it will be really devastating for us. Like, we cannot live without each other, so." She paused. Then she said, "This move was supposed to stabilize things, but it doesn't feel like that. Actually, we don't feel safe at all because we are really worried about eviction. It um—it definitely—it leads to um, more of the hopelessness kind of, a depressed feeling which definitely leads to using more. And a lot more of a f-ck-it attitude."

Patty and Joe then started talking about the similarities between St. Mary's and the newly renovated Lakeshore—the cameras, the fob system, the strict rules about visitors, the regular "wellness checks" by staff, the medical office on their floor—admitting that several friends who had moved in before them had said it was "just like jail." I was struck by how familiar this story was becoming: the endless battles with a rotation of managers, the constant threat of eviction, and the way that young people had to daily navigate building technologies and rules that separated and isolated them from others, when fragile connections to others were the very thing that might keep them alive in the context of mounting overdoses. The difference this time was that Patty and Joe had been expecting something very different. They had been waiting for two years to move back into the Lakeshore. During that time, they had endured living in a place that they hated, struggled with escalating addictions and mental health crises, and undergone multiple long-term hospitalizations. But they had also dreamed: of living in a normal apartment, on the same floor as some of their closest friends, of possibly inviting family members to come and stay with them, and of going back to school.

Patty then disclosed that Joe especially had not been doing well since their move into the Lakeshore. He had developed what they both referred to as "drug-induced schizophrenia" as a result of years of heavy meth use. On several occasions he had been found wandering the halls of the Lakeshore, talking loudly and yelling because he thought he could hear the voices of relatives, could hear them crying out for help. The police had been called on multiple occasions, and Joe had been taken to and held in the hospital on a Mental Health Act apprehension. Patty was attempting to manage the situation as best she could by taking

Joe to see different doctors at a Community Health Center, and the previous day he had started taking risperidone. But they were told at their last medical appointment that Joe's auditory hallucinations could not be managed with psychopharmaceuticals alone. He needed to reduce his meth use. Patty felt strongly that Joe should go home or to detox, and Joe was adamant that he was not ready to take either of those steps. He seemed to be increasingly in his own world. A few weeks later, during one of our rare conversations without Patty present, he told me that he didn't entirely dislike the increasingly hallucinatory world that he was inhabiting. He was scared not of his hallucinations but rather that he and Patty might be evicted, might be separated, and that their separation might cost one or both of them their lives.

After they moved back into the Lakeshore, I watched Patty and Joe's dreams of place collapse with remarkable speed. "We're where they want us to be," Patty told me one day not long after my first visit to the Lakeshore. "This is the end of the line. They have support workers in the building, but what are they there for? Like, to make us clean our rooms and that's it. They give us [harm reduction] supplies. I still have a dealer in the building, and it's like the staff like it that way. It almost seems like they *want* us in our rooms, like, um, alone, using drugs? No one is pushing us to do anything different from that. From here on it's up to us to keep going somewhere," Patty said, but she didn't sound optimistic. It was around this time that she stopped talking about going to treatment.

In a disturbing turn of events, in early 2015 Joe was evicted from the Lakeshore when the police were called to resolve a violent incident between him and Patty. Patty was distraught. She tried desperately to fight the eviction—by insisting that she was not going to press charges against Joe for assaulting her and by attempting to explain that Joe's recent erratic behavior was the result of worsening psychosis. Without her, Patty insisted, Joe would only get worse and could become suicidal. In the end Joe was transferred to a new supportive housing building, where, as Patty predicted, his mental health and drug use worsened until he finally had to be hospitalized under another Mental Health Act apprehension. Patty was moved to a smaller room at the Lakeshore. She began, as she put it, acting crazy as an odd sort of tribute to Joe, yelling and flailing around in the hallway of her new floor just as he had once done, intentionally performing for the camera that was pointed down it. She stopped sleeping. Eventually she was found wandering around downtown with no shoes on. She was picked up by the police and hospitalized under the Mental Health Act for what she later referred to as "a mental breakdown from separation anxiety mixed with depression mixed with bipolar mixed with doing way too many drugs." During this time Patty and Joe broke up.

I continued to visit Patty at the Lakeshore throughout 2015, and Joe occasionally called me or showed up at the field office wanting to talk. It was becoming increasingly difficult to stay in touch with them both. On the one hand, I respected the fact that they were no longer regularly calling me or quickly returning my calls. It was hardly surprising that spending time with me and working on research might no longer interest them, given what was happening in their lives. On the other hand, I wanted to support them if I could because I could see how bad things were getting.

On one occasion in winter 2015 Patty invited me to come and see the smaller room that she had been moved into at the Lakeshore. As we took the elevator together up to her floor, she told me that everything was fine, going well even, but then talked rapidly about how she had deleted her Facebook account and wanted to legally change her name because she believed that people were following her. She was certain the security guard working at a building across the street could see into her room and was watching her. Patty was haunted by her recent experience of being strapped down and forcibly medicated in the hospital, where she also remembered being told by a nurse that she was going to overdose and die. As much as she feared St. Paul's Hospital, she was also in desperate need of care and checked herself into the emergency room on multiple occasions throughout 2015. I regularly observed this tension between the imperative to evade institutionalization and a desire for total care, for a break from feeling and acting crazy, for regular nourishment, and for sleep. By the end of that year, Patty had gotten the impression that she was not allowed at St. Paul's Hospital because of behavioral issues.

When she pushed open the door to her room, I could see that every available surface was covered with a thick layer of detritus: dirty clothing and shoes, old takeout and drink containers, and dozens of uncapped rigs and other drug use paraphernalia. Smeared blood was visible on the pale triangle of floor revealed by the opened door. Keeping rooms in this state was a strategy that a number of those I knew employed to discourage sex work dates from crashing in their rooms for long periods of time and to prevent building staff and various workers from entering. As we stood in the hallway, Patty explained that she had been having difficulty kicking men out, which was her way of beginning to tell me that she had gone back to doing sex work more regularly. She said she was working both out of her room and along the Kingsway stroll in East Vancouver, taking the bus across the city most evenings even though she hated the commute. It was often easier to attract more moneyed clients there, although it was also more dangerous because she had to get into clients' cars.

Patty then abruptly changed the subject by forcefully suggesting we go for coffee at a place nearby. It was below zero out as we walked the few blocks to a coffee shop, carefully stepping over icy cobblestones. Patty wore only a thin blue hoody as she walked beside me because one of her dates had stolen her winter jacket. She had dyed her hair bright red and lost a lot of weight. Patty told me she was really happy with her new look. I could see the blue veins of her face and neck through her pale, translucent skin. I had always thought of Patty as physically solid, formidable even, but that day she seemed small and frail if also beautiful.

Everyone stared as we ordered drinks in the chic coffee bar that Patty had chosen. I suggested that we sit at an open table in the middle of the room, but Patty requested that we take a table in the back, beside a stand where patrons put their dirty dishes and garbage. I took out the photographs that Patty had taken over two years ago, showing her which ones I had had professionally framed for our upcoming exhibit.[17] I complimented her again on her work on the project. Suddenly she became visibly upset. Tears rolled down her face, but she offered no explanation as to why. I reached across the table and put my hand over hers, and we sat in silence for what felt like a long time. She took my hand. Eventually, I asked her how she was feeling about being part of the exhibit. I told her she could pull out if she wanted to. She stared at the table, saying nothing but continuing to hold my hand. I then gently reminded her that the exhibit was not going to be about drug use and addiction but rather about how she and others understood their place in the city. And just as quickly as she became upset, she shifted to excitement. She wiped the tears from her face and started talking about the project: the photos she and Joe had taken, how much she had enjoyed using the different cameras, whom she wanted to invite to the exhibit. By the end of our conversation she had even offered to get everyone together to work on the exhibit on their own time and suggested that we should all go on a fieldtrip to a professional photography exhibit to see an example of what we were trying to create. This was the Patty I knew so well, the young woman who got excited about research and projects. I promised to plan the fieldtrip, but on the day that several of us went to a local art gallery, Patty didn't show up.

Outside the coffee shop that day, she gave me a hug goodbye. As she turned to leave, she said "love you!" just like so many did when they said goodbye to friends. I didn't exactly know why, but it broke my heart that time.

PART 4 NOWHERE

PATTY, SALTWATER CITY, 2017

"Don't die. Don't do too much, don't die, don't die. We just keep telling each other that," Patty said in the spring of 2017. The endless winter (Lupick 2017) of 2016 was over, but the waves of overdose deaths continued, unrelenting. In the heart of the Saltwater City, sirens wailed constantly.[1] Every wall seemed to be crowded with sprawling graffiti and simple etchings memorializing the dead.[2]

THE WILL TO INTERVENE

Vancouver has become an epicenter of North America's current overdose crisis, largely driven by the proliferation of illicitly manufactured synthetic fentanyl, related analogs, and fentanyl-adulterated stimulants in the illicit drug supply (Lupick 2017). The declaration of an overdose public health emergency in 2016 set in motion a churn of new meetings, partnership formations, proposal writing, and guideline development to direct the rapid development, implementation, and scale-up of various services and programs for at-risk populations, including young people who use drugs. The BC Ministry of Mental Health and Addictions was established in 2017 to spearhead these efforts. The creation of a more comprehensive, coordinated, and evidence-based system of substance use services for adolescents and young adults, defined as those twenty-four years of age and under, was identified by the new ministry as a top priority (Government of BC 2019). Over the past several years, the city and province have expanded the number of youth-dedicated residential treatment beds and low-barrier housing sites that incorporate access to mental health and addictions care (VCH 2023c). Community-based harm reduction services such as overdose prevention tents and rooms and the distribution of take-home Naloxone overdose antidote kits also increased dramatically across Greater Vancouver during this period (BC Centre for Disease Control 2021). Two rapid access clinics in downtown Vancouver now provide same-day access to medication-assisted treatment, making it easier to start and restart opioid agonist therapy (OAT; Providence Health

Care 2020; VCH 2023d). In this context I quickly came to realize that while some young people were cycling through these services and on and off OAT at a dizzying rate, others seemed to be moving *around* public health interventions—maneuvers that were arguably no easy feat in the context of a made-in-Vancouver "seek and treat" approach to "treatment as prevention" (Montaner et al. 2006).

Central to ongoing efforts to address the overdose crisis locally was the development of new, evidence-based provincial clinical practice guidelines for the treatment of opioid use disorder, including a youth guideline supplement (BC Centre on Substance Use 2018; BC Centre on Substance Use and BC Ministry of Health 2017). Substance use treatment for adolescents and young adults has traditionally included short-term in-patient withdrawal management (detox) programs and psychosocial treatment interventions (e.g., counselling, cognitive behavioral therapy, contingency management) (Hammond 2016). The new clinical practice guidelines, however, recommend against a treatment strategy involving detox alone and instead strongly endorse the expanded provision of OAT to young people, nested within a broader continuum of care that includes harm reduction services and in- and out-patient psychosocial treatment and various supports (including housing, employment, training, and income assistance).[3] Methadone has long been an established pharmacotherapy for reducing problematic opioid use and attendant harms in Vancouver and elsewhere (Ball and Ross 1991; Nosyk et al. 2014) and has continued to be commonly prescribed to many young people. However, by 2016 Suboxone was the recommended first-line therapy for young people who were diagnosed with opioid use disorder.[4] As my fieldwork progressed additional medication-assisted treatments became available, including slow-release oral morphine (brand name Kadian), a long-acting monthly injectable form of Suboxone (brand name Sublocade), injectable opioid agonist therapy (iOAT; titrated daily witnessed injected doses of diacetylmorphine or hydromorphone), and prescription hydromorphone and dextroamphetamine.[5]

The majority of those I followed were polysubstance users; they used both fentanyl and meth, oftentimes daily, and therefore had been diagnosed with an opioid use disorder, stimulant use disorder, or both. The majority had also been diagnosed with what are referred to as concurrent disorders; that is, they carried with them both substance use disorder diagnoses and one or more psychiatric disorder diagnoses, including bipolar, anxiety, personality, posttraumatic stress (PTSD), and attention-deficit/hyperactivity (ADHD) disorders, depression, and schizophrenia.[6] Many rejected these diagnoses outright; others grappled with whether they were accurate and helpful descriptors of the difficulties they were facing. Regardless, as young people were increasingly put on OAT and other medication-assisted treatments, so too were they increasingly put on psychiatric medications in an effort to provide comprehensive and integrated mental health and addictions care. In particular, over the course of my fieldwork those I followed were increasingly put on second- and third-generation antipsychotics such as aripiprazole, quetiapine, olanzapine, paliperidone, and risperidone to treat recurrent stimulant-induced psychosis alongside one or more of the psychiatric disorders listed above.[7]

While debate continues around the appropriateness of OAT for adolescents and young adults (Fischer et al. 2016), there seemed to be broad support locally for the new clinical practice guidelines and putting greater numbers of young people on OAT, particularly in the context of the overdose emergency.[8] Suboxone, in particular, was tasked with promoting abstinence from illicit opioid use and the protection of life (Stevenson 2014) among at-risk youth.[9] Local physicians and psychiatrists told me that balancing the risks and benefits of prescribing antipsychotic medications was often more difficult. On the one hand, heavy meth use can induce potentially life-threatening hallucinations and paranoia that are similar to those observed in a primary psychotic disorder such as schizophrenia; as stimulant-induced psychotic episodes recur over time, they can become virtually indistinguishable from schizophrenia (Bramness et al. 2012; Fluyau, Mitra, and Lorthe 2019; Glasner-Edwards and Mooney 2014). I was told repeatedly—as were those I followed—that among young people who use meth intensively antipsychotics are simply one of the only tools available to treat recurrent stimulant-induced psychosis and prevent possible damage to the brain. They can help to reduce episodes of agitation, which regularly resulted in eviction from even the most low-barrier supportive housing. On the other hand, stimulant-induced psychotic episodes can be time-limited and resolve without medication (Glasner-Edwards and Mooney 2014). Antipsychotics have various negative side effects, including weight gain, movement disorders (tremors, restlessness, stiffness), agitation and anxiety, sedation and somnolence, and anhedonia (Bramness et al. 2012; Fluyau, Mitra, and Lorthe 2019). These adverse effects may be particularly pronounced among adolescents (McConville and Sorter 2004).

Regardless of potential drawbacks, both OAT and antipsychotics have become increasingly well-integrated into mental health and addictions care for adolescents and young adults across acute, community, and residential treatment settings in Vancouver, including via new intensive case management and outreach teams staffed by physicians, psychiatrists, nurse practitioners, social workers, outreach workers, drug and alcohol counselors, Indigenous Elders, and peer navigators (VCH 2023c).[10] These interdisciplinary teams follow adolescents and young adults as they move between hospital wards, community health clinics, drop-in centers, residential detox, treatment, and recovery sites, shelters, safe houses, and supportive housing buildings located across the city, providing rapid access to and continuity of care alongside other kinds of supports. In addition, addiction medicine consult teams have been created at local hospitals to improve the integration of substance use and mental health care into hospital settings (Providence Health Care 2016).

By 2017 my fieldwork increasingly took me into these care settings. Most of those I had been following over the previous decade—some entering their early thirties by 2017—had long ago aged out of these services, although they had frequented some of them when they were younger. As I spent more time in these places from early 2017, I met many new, younger individuals, most of whom I encountered for much shorter periods of time than those I had been following previously.

SHANE, PASSAGES, 2017

Passages was located in a picturesque residential south Vancouver neighborhood. It was a large house that had been repurposed into a short-term (typically one to two weeks) detox and treatment facility for youth ages thirteen to twenty-four. Current guidelines recommend against these kinds of short-term in-patient stays (BC Centre on Substance Use and BC Ministry of Health 2017) and concerns about the safety and efficacy of this "social" or "community" model in the context of the overdose emergency ultimately led to the closure of Passages in 2022 by the local health authority. However, many young people I knew were attracted to the shorter time frame of the treatment and care they received at Passages (Giang et al. 2020). The thought of entering a longer-term treatment program—particularly in a highly medicalized setting—was, at least initially, overwhelming. Alternatively, going to Passages for anywhere from a few days to a couple of weeks felt like a manageable step toward getting clean. Or it was simply a "break" from the everyday emergencies of addiction in the context of entrenched poverty, homelessness, and unstable housing. Many at Passages were "frequent flyers" who ended up there repeatedly. Young people were court mandated to go to Passages and other places like it; "giving treatment a real try" could be a condition of their parole. Alternatively, like checking yourself into the emergency room, going to Passages was a means of gaining steadier access to nourishment and prioritizing rest and sleep—albeit in a much less institutional setting, which many liked. The building retained its homey feel by design. While individuals were assigned to a particular side of the house on admission based on gender identity, age, and/or intensity of drug use, the doors remained unlocked. There was a large backyard with an apple tree in the middle of it and some plastic deck furniture. The staff at Passages were friendly and laid back; they gave out cigarettes, made grilled cheese sandwiches on request, and were there to talk if individuals were interested.

For many, Passages was where they first heard about what was available to them in terms of treatment programs and other kinds of support. The site was visited daily by nurse practitioners who were part of one of the city's new youth intensive case management teams. These providers would discuss a Suboxone induction with any young person who arrived with the goal of taking even a short-term break from opioid use. Young people were also connected to longer-term residential treatment and recovery programs, day treatment programs, Twelve Step programs, mental health programs, alternative schooling programs, government-subsidized housing programs, outreach programs, and drop-in programs, including the YouthNow "one-stop shop" service hub that delivers comprehensive mental health and addictions care alongside various social services, including recreational activities.

Hearing about these different programs and the anticipation of accessing them after leaving Passages could be a mobilizing experience. "I'm going to start going to the YouthNow drop-in once I get out of here," nineteen-year-old Shane told me in 2017. I had seen him around Passages over the previous few days, but he hadn't been feeling well enough to talk with me. Now he was through the worst of his withdrawal from fentanyl and meth and finally feeling some relief from the Suboxone he had been put on seventy-two hours earlier. We sat together in the living room, talking in low voices while simultaneously binge-watching *Homeland*. Two other young people were shuffling around sleepily in the adjacent kitchen, contemplating food or a cigarette. Shane described the moment when he got to a dose of Suboxone that adequately mediated his cravings as a "light switch." "It seemed like I was feeling miserable, feeling miserable—and then, bam! I was, like, ready to eat five grilled cheese sandwiches all of a sudden," he laughed. Shane had overdosed and been hospitalized less than a week earlier, but like many I encountered at Passages his young age meant that he had recovered remarkably quickly. After only a few days off fentanyl and meth, he already appeared more rested and energized, rapidly tapping his foot on the ground as he spoke.

"[The YouthNow program] apparently has, like, things going on every day, like art programs and outings and activities and classes and stuff like that, that I'm going to start doing. Yeah. One other person here [at Passages], they're like, 'That place [YouthNow] has saved my life.' He was telling me about it. Like, they have, like, just so many different things—everything you need."

Shane eventually added more quietly, "I've had thirteen overdoses in the past *year*, right? If I OD another time, I'm sure I won't come back. So, I'm giving this Suboxone thing a real try and at the moment I'm feeling pretty good about it—about things, in general."

LIVING ON THE EDGE OF CHANGE

"Treatment is incredibly boring," young people told me over and over again. "There's nothing to do there." Certainly, boredom in residential programs and recovery houses was palpable during my fieldwork. I frequently found myself sitting around with them, watching TV until we were all bleary eyed. Many I met in these places agreed that the best way to pass the time was by sleeping as much as possible. In some facilities it was possible to sleep much of the day. In others young people's time was rigorously scheduled.

A typically day could look something like this:

Wake up at 6 or 7 A.M. (depending on if you are on kitchen duty).
Eat breakfast.
Coffee at 8 A.M.
Do your assigned chores.
Take your OAT and other medications.
Go to group therapy (or, in centers for younger people, begin schoolwork).
Smoke break at 10 A.M.
More group therapy or more school.
Eat lunch at 12 P.M.
Do Twelve Step work.
Go for some kind of outing (usually to a fitness center, the library, or a coffee shop).
Eat dinner at 6 P.M.
Go to a Twelve Step meeting.
Lights out at 10 P.M.

Many appreciated how these kinds of strict schedules helped to keep them busy. However, there could also be a monotony to their days. While they could interact with each other in common areas and shared rooms, lively conversations that veered into "war stories" about drug use, dealing, crime, and the dramas of street life were prohibited in all of the residential programs and some of the recovery houses I frequented because of the perception that they could trigger a relapse. Access to mobile phones was also prohibited or restricted in many of these places since contact with those on the outside who were still using drugs was also considered triggering. Young people frequently commented that these kinds of rules left them feeling alone and bored.

But other kinds of affective intensities also circulated in these settings, including a sense of being on the edge of big life changes. While individuals may not always have been engaged in much conversation with other residents, they were regularly drawn into discussions with various workers and providers focused on planning and goal setting for the future. One of the primary mandates of Vancouver's expanding and more coordinated system of youth substance use services is to ensure greater continuity of care and prevent vulnerable individuals from "falling through the cracks" of the multiple systems that they are often traversing, including the government care, criminal justice, healthcare, housing, and frontline service (e.g., shelter) systems (BC Representative for Children and Youth 2015; Government of BC 2019). Across acute, community, and residential treatment settings, a range of workers and providers are implored to work collaboratively with young people on developing "long term, personalized, strengths-based plans" for how to connect them with a range of supports (Government of BC 2019, 13). These supports should then allow them to keep moving forward with goals that include reducing or eliminating illicit drug and alcohol use (or using more safely), addressing mental health challenges, finding housing, reconnecting with school, and gaining employment.

Some entered residential programs with these kinds of goals in mind. Some had to. For many going to residential treatment was a bargaining chip of sorts, something they had to do to satisfy their probation officer or the social worker in charge of their child custody case. However, even for those who did not enter residential programs with these goals in mind, the churn of planning and goal setting that occurred in these places meant that once there many did begin to actively imagine a different kind of future. The lives they began envisioning for themselves often involved better mental and physical health, better opportunities for education, work, and leisure, better housing, and better relationships. This kind of imagining itself generated a sense of momentum, despite chronic boredom.

For people going on Suboxone could energize the planning and goal setting that they were drawn into as their stays in residential programs progressed. The energizing effects of Suboxone were undoubtedly shaped by the growing enthusiasm for this pharmacotherapy on the part of many workers and providers during my fieldwork, which overlapped with the 2017 and 2018 releases of the new clinical guidelines. Beginning around that time young people were increasingly told that Suboxone would not only save but also help to stabilize their lives, allowing other pieces—such as finding a job or finishing school—to fall more easily into place, as one provider put it to me. Taking Suboxone became a way for them to actively invest in different kinds of futures across time and place, including wherever they ended up next.

JESSICA, HORIZONS, 2018

"In treatment, *every single day* is the same thing," sixteen-year-old Jessica told me as she was nearing the end of her six-month stay at Horizons. "You have chores. You have meals. You have group therapy. You have to talk to people about your problems over and over again, but you aren't allowed to talk to other clients [young people] about pretty much anything real that's happened to you. Some people are working on school. But then in some places, they just, like, put you on meds and tell you to rest and watch TV and that's it, right? They don't support you with any of the goals you actually want to work towards." She took a deep breath. "But still, I'm just, like, looking forward to the next thing, which is housing, right? Just having that goal at the end is really helpful to stick it out until I get that call saying, okay, we have housing available for you. I can't wait for that."

While young people's time was far more rigorously scheduled at Horizons than at Passages, the facilities were markedly similar. Horizons was also a large house with a big backyard in a leafy, residential Vancouver neighborhood. It was comfortably furnished and had a homey feel. The walls of the entryway were decorated with colorful artwork made by former youth clients. Much of this artwork evoked a sense of transformation from feeling sad and adrift to feeling happy and motivated.

By this point in her stay Jessica was allowed to leave Horizons for outings during the evenings and on weekends, and I had driven us to a nearby Starbucks for coffee. We didn't know each other well. We had chatted only briefly a couple of times at Horizons while I was visiting another person there. A staff member at Horizons had told me that Jessica had heard about the research I was doing and was eager to talk to me. On the drive to Starbucks, I got the impression that she was eager for an outing of any kind. She told me that she had a very difficult relationship with her birth family and her former foster parents and was trying to distance herself from an ex-boyfriend who was still using fentanyl. She had therefore not had many visitors beyond her "workers," who also took her out for coffee when they came by.

Jessica told me that she had been on Suboxone throughout her entire stay at Horizons and it was going really well. "I'm taking my Suboxone each day and I'm just, like, really trying to stay focused and keep going with, like, my plans for the future," she said, before admitting that she had thought about leaving Horizons dozens of times. "It's incredibly, *incredibly* hard to, like, keep going in treatment, when you're, like, so bored but also overwhelmed and, like, really missing your boyfriend. But, like, *amazingly*, I'm still here. And now it's, like, almost the end," she chuckled. "I really did it, this time. Somehow, I did, like, stay? Part of that is because of Suboxone, I think. It's really helped me."

Several weeks later at a different Starbucks nearby our field office in downtown Vancouver, Jessica told me about how things were going now that she had finished the program at Horizons and moved into her housing. She was on a Youth Agreement, which meant that she received a monthly subsidy for rent and other necessities that allowed her to live independently (although she was under nineteen years of age) while she pursued returning to school. Freshly made up and wearing a stylish outfit, her appearance, tone, and posture all exuded energy and optimism. She continued to attribute much of her success to staying on Suboxone.

"I've had zero cravings [for opiates]," Jessica said happily. "And, like, I feel so, like, *productive* on Suboxone. It just, like, helps with that—with keeping going—I think. I've just, like, been really keeping myself busy, handing out my resume. Just for basic shitty retail jobs, but still. I'm planning on going back to school in the fall, and I think there's just no way that would be possible without the Suboxone."

After a while she added more cautiously, "I just hope that I can, like, keep going? At treatment, they told me, like, 'Good luck, and we're here for you if you relapse'—like they are *expecting* that to happen, right? Which is not, like, something I want to hear. It's like, I don't want to be a drug addict for my whole life, you know? Don't, like, expect me to fail."[11]

FILLING THE HOURS

Young people explained to me repeatedly that staying off drugs and pursuing the futures they wanted for themselves meant "just keeping going" and "filling the hours." Periods of sitting around with nothing to do were feared (Mains 2012) because they could fuel a troubling sense that one was going nowhere despite daily efforts to keep moving forward. When this sense of stagnation overwhelmed them, the result was almost always relapse. To avoid this, young people attempted to construct elaborate daily schedules, describing to me in detail how they kept themselves busy each day while avoiding the people, places, and things that could trigger a relapse. They tried to keep *moving*, spending hours and hours riding different SkyTrain lines or walking and biking across the city and its suburbs. One young man I knew spent almost all of his waking hours dancing to music, in his room and outside the public art gallery downtown, in an effort to keep himself off meth.

OAT and antipsychotic medications could powerfully intersect with a feared sense of stagnation. Going on these pharmacotherapies lessened the daily frenzied rhythms of addiction in the sense that young people no longer had to navigate the threat of withdrawal and psychosis with the same intensity. While this was a tremendous relief, they often found themselves at a loss for how to fill the hours in the absence of much of the drama that had filled their days previously. Instead of drama, daily witnessed dosing requirements meant that, for those on OAT, each and every day came to be marked by the repetitiveness of trips to the pharmacy or a knock on the door of their supportive housing room. In addition, methadone and Kadian can both cause sedation and weight gain, particularly when taken at the doses required to moderate cravings for fentanyl. Drowsiness and weight gain are also common side effects of a number of second-generation antipsychotics. Many described feeling increasingly lethargic while they were on these pharmacotherapies. They hated the weight that they had gained and yet could not seem to stop themselves from sleeping the days away. They found it tremendously difficult to motivate themselves and get things done.

The affective intensities of Suboxone could be markedly different. Several young people commented that Suboxone not only mediated cravings but also gave them a heightened ability to get going each day. Suboxone made them feel productive and helped them to keep busy. Despite this, most of those I knew preferred methadone and Kadian to Suboxone because of the euphoric—if also sedating—effects of the former (Giang et al. 2020). To wake themselves up from their OAT and antipsychotic medications many used meth at least once but often multiple times a day, riding endless waves of mania and sedation, momentum and stagnation.

SHANE, DOWNTOWN, 2017

"I've been, like, so busy. But I'm so tired," Shane admitted to me in late 2017, a few weeks before he stopped picking up his daily witnessed dose of Suboxone at the pharmacy and relapsed on fentanyl.

After spending two weeks at Passages earlier that year, Shane completed a three-month residential program at Horizons. While it was possible to stay at Horizons for longer, following a series of altercations between Shane and another client, the decision was made to move him to a second-stage recovery house for men ages nineteen and older located in a suburb of Greater Vancouver.[12]

"It was kind of bullshit the way I ended up leaving Horizons," Shane told me when I visited him at his new house. We sat in the large, breezy backyard while he chain-smoked cigarettes and picked at the paint that was peeling off the weathered wooden picnic table. "But they still threw me a big party and everything for finishing the three months, which was pretty cool. I did really try there, actually. And when I left I actually, like, felt super motivated and like things could be different this time. I was still like, yeah! Rehab is awesome! Suboxone is awesome!"

Across my fieldwork, recovery houses in Greater Vancouver varied enormously in terms of living environments and the kinds of supports provided.[13] Some were highly informal and notorious for open drug dealing and use, leading many young people to compare them to crack shacks and "flophouses"; others featured hour-by-hour programming that usually revolved around group therapy sessions, Twelve Step meetings, work, meals, and chores. Many were somewhere in between. Shane found himself at a decent one, but he struggled to maintain the sense of momentum he had found while in residential treatment at Passages and Horizons. In his recovery house, he felt the familiar threat of inertia.

"I've been going to Twelve Step meetings," he told me that day in the backyard. "That's basically something I do just to fill my days so I'm not sitting around alone doing nothing and, like, having cravings. It just really helps to get out of this house every day and go to meetings and then meet up with people after for a coffee. But I can feel my energy, like, draining away, or something. Somehow that's happening again."

A few weeks later Shane came into our field office, lay down on a row of chairs in our waiting area, and told me that he didn't think he could get back up. He mumbled that, in addition to using fentanyl, he was also at the end of a weeklong meth binge. His plan was to rest at our office for a while and then walk the few blocks to St. Paul's Hospital where he would check himself into the psychiatric ward. "My mind doesn't feel right," he said repeatedly. "It's on the verge on snapping, I think."

In an email he wrote to me around a month later, Shane explained that he had relapsed on meth while in the recovery house. Using meth was a means of staving off a relapse on fentanyl and maintaining the momentum he needed to continue attending daily Twelve Step meetings and connecting with his sponsor. In the end, however, a much-feared sense of stagnation came in the form of regular doses of antipsychotic medication during a weeklong stay in the psychiatric ward.

STALLS AND DEAD ENDS

Ideally, young people moved directly from short-term residential programs like Passages to longer-term residential programs like Horizons and then directly into some form of safe and supportive housing (e.g., a family, foster care, or group home if they were under nineteen years of age, and transitional or recovery housing if they were over nineteen).[14] Those between the ages of sixteen and twenty-six who were (or were formerly) involved with the Ministry of Children and Family Development were eligible for a few different provincial independent living programs, which provided a monthly subsidy for market rental housing, education, and training, as well as other kinds of supports (e.g., weekly visits from a youth worker to assist with building life skills such as grocery shopping, cooking, cleaning, managing money, and communicating with landlords) (Government of BC 2021a, 2021b).

However, these kinds of plans often fell through, stalled, or dead-ended. Program wait lists and time lags between placements and an inability to secure market rental and government-subsidized housing often led to periods of street-based homelessness, couch surfing, and temporary shelter or safehouse stays. Young people frequently commented that once their time was up at residential treatment they were often right back at square one. This left many with the sense that no matter how hard they tried, they couldn't *get anywhere*.

Housing unavailability is shaped by various factors, not the least of which is Vancouver's exorbitant housing market and rental costs. Supportive housing is limited and often inappropriate for those who are attempting to maintain abstinence because of the volume of drug use and dealing in many of these settings. Several treatment program managers commented to me that foster care, group home, and independent living placements for adolescents and young adults seem to be increasingly scarce, as homeowners make the decision to convert basement suites to much more lucrative market or Airbnb rentals rather than take in a young person in government care or rent to someone on social assistance.

In many cases young people were adamant that they could not return to chaotic family homes, even when the ministry deemed these settings safe.

Fragmented institutional and housing trajectories meant that the sense of momentum and promise generated by the churn of planning and goal setting in residential treatment and recovery programs could quickly dissipate. Most also continued to endure the quiet ravages of inadequate monthly income assistance payments and entrenched poverty, which frequently left them sitting around with nothing to do. They aged out of the services and programs they had once been so excited about accessing, deepening isolation, boredom, and stagnation.

Under these kinds of structural pressures, imaginaries of different, better futures and a commitment to staying on Suboxone or another form of OAT often collapsed. Some did seem willing to try and keep moving forward with treatment one way or another, even as they moved in and out of shelters, hospital wards, and residential programs, experienced numerous slips, relapses, and overdoses, and went on and off Suboxone or another form of OAT at a dizzying rate. Others, however, were not able or willing to keep going. Many became engaged in another kind of seemingly endless cycle of withdrawal and return beyond that which characterizes addiction. They withdrew from the treatment programs that they had engaged with previously and then were drawn back into the system at regular moments of crisis, usually when they required shelter or hospitalization.

LULA, WENONAH HOUSE, 2016

At the end of 2011 and the start of 2012, Lula attended a six-month residential treatment program in another province. This was, as she put it, a "do-or-die, last-ditch effort" to regain custody of the one-year-old daughter she shared with Jeff by that time. The plan had been to get out of downtown, to get away, so that she could focus on herself and her recovery without the distraction of her friends and in particular Jeff.

During her pregnancy and immediately following the birth of her daughter in early 2011, Lula had also twice attended Fern Grove, a Vancouver-based residential treatment program for pregnant individuals and families. She told me she was "kicked out" both times for failing to follow the rules. While Lula was highly committed to remaining abstinent from crack during her first pregnancy and following the birth of her daughter, she seemed utterly unable to commit herself to a separation from Jeff and her friends who were continuing to use drugs intensively. Her inability to separate from Jeff—who seemed to have no intention of stopping using drugs—resulted in the swift loss of custody of their daughter following her birth in 2011, even though Lula largely remained abstinent from crack. When she half-heartedly reentered Fern Grove without custody of her daughter, she again found herself bored and alone, with "nothing to fill her time with." Her anxiety grew until she "just couldn't hold it all together anymore." She took off to see Jeff and her friends, despite warnings from staff that this would mean being asked to leave the program and permanently losing custody of her daughter.

Lula then lived with Jeff for two months in the Lakeshore Hotel. While staying at the Lakeshore with Jeff, Lula relapsed on crack, and she and Jeff began fighting constantly and viciously about what they did or did not need to do to change their lives and regain custody of their daughter. Their time together at the Lakeshore ended when Jeff went to jail on yet another charge related to their violent disputes, and Lula decided to give residential treatment a "real try." The two broke up, and with the support of her parents Lula flew out of the city and away from Jeff to attend residential treatment at the end of 2011. She told me that she wasn't exactly sure why she had relapsed as soon as she got home from the six-month program, but she hated herself for being one of those moms who wasn't able to give up drugs for her child.

Lula briefly considered going back to the same treatment program, but instead a new boyfriend had introduced her to meth, which quickly got her off crack (Fast et al. 2014). On meth, her life stabilized in certain ways.[15] She no longer had to steal all day to pay for hit after hit of crack, because a point of meth was relatively cheap and could last twenty-four hours. Treatment suddenly seemed irrelevant. Lula told me that the downside to daily meth use was that it exacerbated her schizoaffective disorder and depression. The quetiapine, lamotrigine, and venlafaxine that she had been taking since early adolescence didn't work as well when she was using meth intensively, and she regularly stopped taking them. Despite the volatility of their relationship, Jeff more than anyone else helped Lula to manage her mental health as she continued to use meth. He told her repeatedly not to listen to the voices in her head and that no one was out to get her. Perhaps that was one of the things that brought them back together, even as they fairly regularly tried to move on with other romantic partners.

By the end of 2012, Lula became pregnant for the second time. She had been moved into a women-only supportive housing building called Wenonah House that included pregnancy- and parenting-related services and mental health and addictions care, while Jeff had been moved into the Greystone Hotel (another supportive housing building) because the Lakeshore Hotel was undergoing renovation. Unlike most supportive housing buildings, Lula's suite at Wenonah House had a full kitchen and bathroom. And while she hated the building rules as much as anyone else I knew, she ended up staying there for five years, despite permanently loosing custody of both her children, largely for refusing to break off her relationship with Jeff.

Lula became pregnant for a third time in late 2016, and the sequence of events that had occurred with her previous pregnancies and births largely repeated themselves with devastating consequences. I visited Lula regularly throughout her third pregnancy and watched with a growing sense of unease as she repeatedly ignored warnings from her social worker and Wenonah House staff that if she did not distance herself from Jeff (who was essentially living in her room even though he was allowed to sleep over only two nights per week) she was at risk of losing custody of her child following the birth. She was also at risk of losing her housing. While my close relationship with both Lula and Jeff made me feel conflicted about offering my own warnings, Lula's desire to maintain custody of her child this time ultimately led me to add my voice to those of the social worker and housing staff. I told Lula whenever we saw each other that if she did not distance herself from Jeff, I did not think she would be allowed to keep her baby.

"I know, I know, I know—I'm going to do it [break up with Jeff]," Lula told me each time I raised the issue. And yet as the clock on her pregnancy ran down (Knight 2015), Jeff continued to sleep over every night. Each time I visited them, I noticed with alarm the large pile of syringes that littered the floor beside his side of the mattress. But I also came to recognize that Jeff was Lula's only consistent source of support throughout this pregnancy. He brought her food and cooked for her almost every single day, helped her up from and down onto her mattress as her belly grew, and calmed her down again and again when she became overwhelmed with anxieties about the future. Lula's romantic relationship with Jeff was also at the center of her moral universe (Zigon 2013). The third baby was not Jeff's, and yet he had "majorly stepped up" to take care of Lula during this pregnancy, a gesture that ignited the moral world they shared and bound Lula even more tightly to him. Jeff had done the right thing when the baby's father had not. Jeff was there for her when no one else was. Lula therefore could not and would not envision getting through this pregnancy without Jeff, even as the mounting anxieties she was facing must have been partially shaped by a realization that the path she was on would almost certainly result in the losses of custody and housing. At the same time Lula was highly ambivalent about staying in her current housing, despite the fact that Wenonah House was one of the only supportive housing buildings that included specialized programing for pregnant individuals and families.

"Once the baby is here, I don't want to be in a place with harm reduction supplies and stuff," she told me one day as we sat on her bed together. "I don't want my kid to see that, and to see people using and stuff. And, I don't want the temptation of going back to using, which is what I associate this place with."

Lula picked at the red yarn hair of a Cabbage Patch Kid doll that she still occasionally slept with, not making eye contact with me. She was at the end of her second trimester and feeling tired and uncomfortable. Beyond the fatiguing effects of pregnancy, she also seemed weighed down by the enormity of the situation she was faced with. She told me that she had been spending most of her time sleeping and finding it hard to get out of bed. Cognizant of this, I was nevertheless attempting to gently but frankly talk with her about the things that needed to happen to get custody of her child this time. Lula admitted that she was hoping her parents would help her to find and pay for market rental housing, even though they had not seen each other in months and had grown distant. I got the sense that they were not happy about the third pregnancy. I studied the walls of her room, covered with pictures of her kids, posters of pop stars, postcards sent to her by her parents while they were on vacation (and a couple from me), and a half dozen memorial announcements for friends who had passed away. In the middle of it all was a printout of the resident's creed from the six-month treatment program she had attended in 2011 and 2012. It read,

> I have come here in search of myself. Confused and afraid, I have led my life in the shadow of drugs. I have rejected all who cared for me and loved me. I had become a stranger to my family. Guilt, lies and hurt became my most intimate companions, drugs and alcohol my most cherished friends. I belonged nowhere and to no one. I felt desperately alone.

> Here at last, I have found true friends. I no longer need to be the giant of my dreams or the dwarf of my fears. I am allowed to be genuine, to express my emotions. My friends act as a mirror for me, our common quest heals me. The strengths, love and dreams that now live within me have become beacons for my life. From here I will go forth, whole once more, self-aware, confident and assured, never to live in the shadows again.

I asked Lula why she kept the resident's creed on her wall after all these years, and she told me it comforted her. She said she read it to herself most days. I asked her if she was planning on trying to go back to Fern Grove before the baby was born or afterward. Although Lula had told me that she had been mostly abstinent from meth throughout her pregnancy, I knew that social workers almost always insisted that mothers with a history of substance use complete some kind of treatment program before being granted custody of their children. But Lula was highly ambivalent about the idea of treatment.

"I already know all that treatment stuff," she shrugged, tossing the doll aside. She grimaced as she adjusted herself on the bed. "I've given that a try and it didn't really get me anywhere. I ended up right back living in an SRO [Wenonah House] downtown for drug users, which is what tends to happen to pretty much everyone—that I know, at least." She paused. "And I guess maybe it's also about the fact that I don't have anyone to go with? I don't want to go to treatment on my own." I heard this again and again. Living on the edge of change—reading the resident's creed each day, longing to be reunited with children or to maintain custody of a new child—was one thing. But to actually make such a big change,

Lula wanted—needed—to be with someone: a romantic partner, a friend, a family member. The resident's creed on her wall talked about the loneliness and isolation of addiction, and yet, like so many others, Lula told me she had never felt so lost and alone—and bored—as when she was in treatment.

Suddenly, Lula was in tears. "Right now, I think I'm at the lowest point in my life," she said. "Even though I'm not using [meth]. And it's just like, when am I going to start digging myself out of this hole? When am I going to start moving *forward*? I want to keep this baby, I want to be a good mom. I'm hoping that this pregnancy is, like, a blessing in disguise, for me to be able to move on to living, like, the normal life that I've been dreaming of for so many years, you know?" She wiped her face with the sleeve of her sweatshirt. "I'm so tired of that old life. I really can't keep doing what I've been doing, and yet I keep on doing it, going back to it. I'm just like, why do I keep on doing it? Why can't I just stop?" Lula took a deep, shaky breath. "And I keep coming back to, well, if I do stop that life, what am I going to do with my time? How am I going to fill my time? What is my life *actually* going to look like? You know?"

EVERYTHING WE NEED, CARLY AND CONNOR, 2013

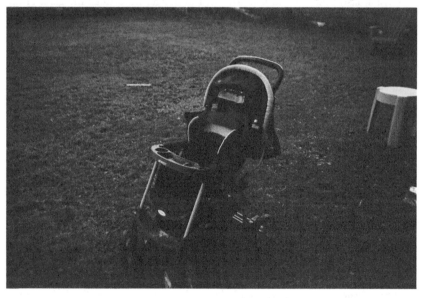

A CHURN OF INTERVENTION

Like the public health emergencies that preceded it, the overdose emergency has generated an affective churn of intervention across the care assemblage. There were moments when those I followed became swept up in the momentum of this churn, and the goal setting and planning exercises that are increasingly integral to both in- and out-patient programs designed to treat those diagnosed with substance use and concurrent psychiatric disorders. In these moments, treatment could seem to hold out the promise of a different, better future: a future in which it was possible to finish school, get a job, find a nicer place to live, enter into healthier relationships, and, for a number of young people, be a good parent. However, this sense of momentum existed alongside the sense of stagnation that was generated by plans that regularly fell through, stalled, or dead-ended. The churn of intervention—which encompassed everything from substance use and psychiatric disorder diagnoses to pitiful monthly social assistance payments and undesirable supportive housing—ensnared many in rhythms of starts and stops that didn't seem to get them anywhere, generating deep ambivalence toward the care assemblage.[16] This was evident both among those I had known for years and among the new group of younger individuals that I began encountering. It led some to increasingly evade or refuse many programs. Instead, they carved out zones of the city where the use of fentanyl and meth could generate a sense of momentum that was hooked not on futures but on the sensorial possibilities of the now.[17]

RAYMOND, DOWNTOWN, 2017

I ran into twenty-year-old Raymond on the street in downtown Vancouver only hours after he had left the hospital against medical advice (AMA). Raymond is Anishinaabe First Nations and moved from Winnipeg to Vancouver when he was fourteen to reconnect with an uncle who was living in the Downtown Eastside. I first met him in 2016 at a safe house where he spent a few days after being hospitalized for an overdose. He had just aged out of government care and been released from jail and was moving between short stints in safe houses and periods of street-based homelessness. He loved hockey and had longed to play as a kid. When he was younger he had enjoyed and excelled in school when he was able to attend. His dad had been killed in a gang-related incident only a few years previously, and Raymond himself had a long history of gang involvement and participation in serious crime. Since he was twelve he had been in and out of group homes, juvenile detention centers, and jails located across multiple provinces. He was pretty sure that it was while he was in jail in Saskatoon that he had managed to finish high school—although it might have been while he was in a group home there. These places were often impossible to distinguish in his memories of the past.

Raymond struck me as at once incredibly tough and remarkably vulnerable. That day in 2017 he was wandering around alone, his plastic hospital bracelet still around his wrist. He told me that earlier that morning he suffered an overdose that could not be reversed with six shots of Narcan. It was his twentieth overdose during the previous year. As we sat on a park bench he explained wearily, "In the last year, this is when I started overdosing, right, because I just—things are not going to get any better in my life, right? So, I just started using more and more, you know? I was—I was afraid, you know, of the future, afraid of the past and afraid of the present, right? You know, too scared to kill yourself, but I was close to death each time. I am close to death."

I immediately began trying to talk Raymond into letting me take him somewhere for further medical attention or so that he could at least talk to someone. "What about Elder Neil [from one of the intensive case management teams]?" I suggested, in an attempt to connect Raymond with a more "culturally safe" model of care (First Nations Health Authority 2015). Those I knew, whether Indigenous or not, often told me how much they loved Elder Neil. But Raymond just stared at the ground, slowly kicking at the gravel with his shoe. I then brought up the idea of a stay at Passages.

"Residential treatment places are where a lot of angry Native kids get put," he told me sharply. Raymond pulled the hood of his sweatshirt over his head and got up to go. "Foster care, group homes, jail—it's all the same," he muttered. Those I knew often expressed this sentiment, no matter how tirelessly those on the front lines worked to make treatment programs "low barrier," "youth friendly," and culturally safe. At this point I knew better than to bring up OAT. Following one of his earlier hospitalizations Raymond had been put on methadone to treat his opioid use disorder and long-acting injectable paliperidone to treat meth-related psychosis. The methadone had helped with the dopesickness (painful opioid withdrawal symptoms) when he got stuck without fentanyl. But he quickly hated the way that methadone combined with the paliperidone to make him feel like he had "no feelings" and sleep all day.

"The antipsychotic shot they put you on is completely debilitating," he had told me previously. "It basically takes your whole life away. You can't really get out of bed, you can't work, you can't have a girlfriend—like, you can't participate in a conversation properly. My girlfriend and I fought constantly when I was on that."

While he was on methadone and paliperidone, Raymond used meth and alcohol to wake himself up and "feel some emotions." Now that he was off both he seemed to be actively avoiding any service setting where he might be put back on either. Instead, he used cannabis intensively to mediate withdrawal symptoms and cravings when he decided he needed to curb his drug use or was dopesick (Paul et al. 2020). He used fentanyl to come off meth when he felt vulnerable to an episode of psychosis, and meth to come off fentanyl when he got tired of waking up dopesick (Fast et al. 2014). Raymond also occasionally talked about going home to Winnipeg as a way of taking a break from drugs altogether. More often he joked that jail could be a particularly effective form of treatment, assuring me that he would be back there at some point—probably sooner than later.

I feebly offered Raymond the food I had in my bag and told him that he could call me later if he needed help. He replied more forcefully, "No, no—I'm going to catch the SkyTrain out of here [downtown Vancouver] now. Go get some dope. Have some fun. Get into trouble." Raymond's most recent probation conditions included various red zone restrictions and an order to remain in Vancouver. These were intended to curtail his movements through and in and out of the city, but he insisted on staying mobile.

"Where can I find you?" I asked, somewhat desperately. "I just want to check in to make sure you're okay."

"You can't," he laughed. "I don't stay in one spot. I'm always moving from place to place, right? *Making distance.* I'm everywhere. I'm everywhere." And with that he took off down the street without looking back.

THE COLONIAL PRESENT

Tanana Athabascan scholar Dian Million (2013, 46) has argued that colonialism itself is a "felt, affective relationship." It is a "residue of common experience sensed but not [always] spoken" (Berlant 2011, 65), particularly in ways that fit neatly with medicalized imaginaries of disorder, treatment, and healing. Local Indigenous scholars, activists, and organizations have demonstrated how disproportionate rates of addiction, overdose, and other harms among Indigenous people in Vancouver and BC are powerfully constituted by the colonial past and present (First Nations Health Authority 2017; Goodman et al. 2017; Lavalley et al. 2018; Martin and Walia 2019; Pearce et al. 2015; Turpel-Lafond 2020)—as are their proposed solutions. Residential treatment and OAT echo colonial logics of control, even as providers increasingly work to ensure that programs are culturally safe.[18]

The young Indigenous people I knew rarely spoke to me (a white settler researcher) directly about how being Indigenous and the legacy of colonialism shaped their drug use and engagement (or lack thereof) with state-sponsored systems and services. Instead, their words to me often seemed to reflect a felt knowledge of how the past can weigh on the present and the future to create a sense of stagnation that cannot be easily addressed by even the most culturally safe treatment programs, as we might hope. Their refusal of residential treatment as just another in a long line of places where "angry Native kids get put" carried the residue of intergenerational experiences. These include the systematic dispossession of land and forced poverty, one hundred years of residential schooling, the Sixties and Millennium Scoops (throughout which thousands of First Nations, Métis, and Inuit children have been taken from their families and placed into foster care or put up for adoption), racist policing and high rates of incarceration, and successive waves of pathologization and containment related to public health emergencies such as tuberculosis, HIV, and suicide (Stevenson 2014).

The relationship between past, present, and future deepened ambivalence toward treatment among some of the Indigenous young people I knew and informed moments of refusal (Simpson 2014): refusals to wait for the ambulance after an overdose, to go to or stay in the hospital or residential treatment center, to take OAT, and to be knowable and countable as "just another Indigenous youth overdose death." These moments of refusal or "turning away" (Coulthard 2014; Fanon 2008) from the state-sponsored churn of intervention were almost never explicitly politicized in the ways that Audra Simpson (2014) describes in her ethnography of the Kahnawà:ke Mohawks—or at least those politics were rarely made visible to me. However, they were generative of other lines of potential, including an impulse to be everywhere and therefore not so easily surveilled, tracked, counted, or contained.

Instead of looking to state-sponsored systems and services to engender a sense of forward momentum in their lives, many young Indigenous people I knew often gestured to the imminent possibilities of intensive drug use, getting into trouble (Jervis, Spicer, and Manson 2003), and geographic mobility.[19] These were alternative ways of binding themselves to life beyond the care assemblage, even as they brought them into close proximity with death (Goodfellow 2008). Being everywhere perhaps mirrored the transience that many had experienced while growing up, cycling through foster care and group homes, juvenile detention centers, jails, and treatment facilities. But it was also a way of being in the world that refused detainment, thereby perhaps engendering a greater sense of power and safety.

AARON, FIELD OFFICE, 2017

By spring 2017 Aaron was using much less meth and was wired to fentanyl. He was continuing to avoid alcohol following his mom's death from alcoholism in 2009. He told me that he had started doing fentanyl because everybody else he knew was doing it and because there didn't seem to be any good reason not to do it. He described his fentanyl use as "out of control" but was adamant about not wanting to access any form of substance use care.

"I don't want to go to detox. I don't want to go to treatment," he told me tiredly, but firmly. I had been in the middle of explaining to him how my research had recently shifted to focus on how young people engaged with these kinds of programs across time. Aaron's visit to the field office that day was unexpected. I had not seen much of him since he and Laurie had broken up almost one year earlier. I knew that he continued to hate the place where he was living and spent most of his time in the Beachwood Hotel, a privately owned SRO that was becoming increasingly notorious for crime and violence.[20] I had run into him a few times in the Downtown Eastside, where he regularly sold shoplifted meat, cheese, brand-name jeans, and other merchandise. While the police regularly tried to push Aaron into the city-sanctioned street market (Downtown Eastside Street Market Society 2014), he usually preferred to sell his wares on the streets, spreading them out on a patch of sidewalk. Despite regular involvement in various illegal income generation schemes across the years I had known him, Aaron was masterful at avoiding charges and jail time. In 2017 he was limiting his participation in the merch economy to selling stuff for others or engaging in an elaborate series of purchases and trades to procure a few choice items—Hello Kitty backpacks, designer sunglasses—that he could sell for a profit. He adamantly refused to do any shoplifting himself, an activity that sent many other young people to jail repeatedly.

Sitting together in the office that day, I asked Aaron whether he had been using any of the overdose prevention sites springing up across the downtown core, including one that was started by several prominent activists connected to the street market (Lupick 2017). Aaron replied curtly that he "didn't pay attention to any of that stuff and didn't need to" because he had never overdosed. His annoyance at where I was leading our conversation—toward a discussion of various services and programs—was palpable, and I wondered if he was going to cut it short. Instead, he suddenly brought up the center in Alberta where he had been forced to live for several years during his adolescence, referring to it by name for the first time. During a conversation several years earlier he had referred to it as a rehabilitation center. This time he was adamant that it was a "treatment facility." When I was able to later look it up online, I learned that it was a long-term residential facility for "complex high-risk youth," including those experiencing addiction.

"There were a lot of Native kids there," Aaron said flatly. "And I wasn't allowed—I had to stay within—within arm's reach of a staff person. We only left the center to go into the city, like, a couple of times maybe. I finally got away from there by punching some kid out, because that treatment program, they don't accept violence, right? So they sent me back to Whitehorse."

He paused. "So, yeah. I don't like going to treatment. I don't like going to jail. I don't want to access any of that." Then he looked me straight in the eye and added pointedly, "I don't want to think about it." We changed the subject for a while.

Aaron told me on different occasions that he did whatever he could to avoid experiences of (re)institutionalization in supportive housing buildings, jail, and residential treatment centers, where both a sense of being controlled and long stretches of sitting around with nothing to do could surface painful and dangerous memories. Memories of being ripped away from family, of loved ones who were gone, and of violence experienced, witnessed, and perpetrated. Memories that could cause him to lash out in violence, fall apart, or go crazy. There are important differences between these places, of course. But for Aaron and so many others they could often feel interchangeable, and because of that they were places to evade at all costs.

The drugs also helped with not thinking too much about the past or future. "The dope keeps things off my mind, right?" Aaron explained, as he finished off the extra-large coffee loaded with sugar, cream, and some kind of marshmallow candy that I had bought him at the 7-Eleven across the street. "I'm not trying to quit. I like doing drugs." But after a while he continued thoughtfully, "If I do stop the dope, I'm not going to get help. I don't *want* help. I'll do it on my own, just like I did before with the drinking, right? Because I'll have more of a chance of relapsing if I get help."

I had heard this sentiment expressed many times, but I still asked him what he meant.

"None of that treatment stuff actually *works*. Like if you go to treatment and stuff, you're taking yourself away from your environment, going where there's not really—like, as soon as you get back, you're going to want dope and relapse. That's just taking a break, I guess. That's weaker." He continued, "But if you just stay in your environment, and try and deal with the problem yourself, once you get through it you'll have that choice to not go back to the dope, because you've been around it the whole time and you've quit while you're around it. That's showing strength in yourself."

Aaron did not seem to believe that entering residential treatment would ultimately take him somewhere better—in fact, it could take him to the worst, most frightening parts of his own mind. He firmly believed that once the program was over he would be back living at some supportive housing building or other, where it was neither possible nor preferable to stay off meth and fentanyl unless he decided that was how he wanted things to be.

LIVING WITH DEATH

I watched as young people's possibilities increasingly unfolded through but also around treatment. Even as the geography of overdose prevention sites, patrols, and outreach teams expanded to cover more and more of the interstitial spaces where drug use takes place in Greater Vancouver, they continued to carve out hidden spaces for themselves: bridge underpasses, uninhabited beaches, and semiforested areas where they camped alone or in small groups to avoid drawing the attention of workers, providers, and police. There were also those who carved out these spaces right up against those of intensive intervention: inside a handful of privately owned SROs, along alleyways, and in tent cities and well-hidden camps in downtown Vancouver.

In these places young people frequently acknowledged that they were "living on the edge of" or "with death," as those who had overdosed and been brought back multiple times sometimes described it. The momentum of fentanyl and meth use was simultaneously a source of fun, terror, and loss in the context of a toxic drug supply and the other forms of everyday violence that marked their lives. Most of those I knew had long ago lost count of the number of friends and family members they had lost to fatal overdoses. And yet in these lives lived alongside death (Stevenson 2014), the intensive use of fentanyl and meth had a desired kind of momentum that was hooked not on futures but on the sensorial possibilities of the now. The frenzied daily rhythms and geographies of addiction meant that there would always be another all-consuming mission, interpersonal drama, and high on the horizon.[21]

Young people were sometimes captured by the systems they were trying to avoid. Consequently, they learned to jump out of ambulances before they reached the hospital or leave AMA when they ended up there after overdosing. They learned to say, in a tired but firm tone, "No, I'm not interested in treatment," on those occasions when they woke up in the hospital or were forced to access care for blood-borne infections like hep C and endocarditis. And sometimes they also pushed firmly against continued involvement in my research, which they knew was increasingly focused on treatment and futurity by design.

LULA AND JEFF, FIELD OFFICE, 2017

"In this past year, I've lost about thirty friends down here," Lula told me at the end of 2017. She, Jeff, and I were sitting in the field office. "I counted. And I think I even had an overdose, recently. I went down, and the ambulance came and everything, but in the end I didn't want to go to the hospital. Because even the meth is contaminated with fentanyl now, I saw recently—there was a [health authority] announcement about that, warning us—"

"A lot of people in my building have died. I hear people overdosing in my hallway," Jeff cut in. He did this less now that he was primarily using fentanyl but still sometimes talked over Lula while the three of us were together. "Like, in our buildings, okay, you *can't* have guests on Welfare Day. So you feel really unsafe because no one is going to be there to save you from an overdose. It's like playing Russian roulette."

Lula shot Jeff an angry look for cutting her off. She continued more forcefully, "They want us in our rooms using alone so that we can die alone. I'm on so many housing lists but I don't want to go to supportive housing, I don't want to go to modular housing [another, oftentimes temporary form of housing introduced by the City of Vancouver during the later years of my fieldwork] because that's, like, a death camp." She continued, "I'm just sick and tired of watching my friends drop like flies around me. Everyday I'm wondering, who's next? Am *I* next? And the thing is, my friends who have died, they're just, like, a statistic to the government. Some of my friends have been saying, 'It's population control,' or like, people are talking about 'fentrification.' Because it's like, what did they do when the Olympics came? They wanted to push us away, get us out of sight for the tourists. But it's like, now they're slowly killing us. It's one big genocide. All these people dying is part of the plan."

While I had seen Lula and Jeff frequently throughout Lula's pregnancy in 2016 and 2017, I hadn't seen much of them since the baby was born earlier that year. I knew from a few sporadic phone conversations with Lula that following the birth of her daughter she had spent six weeks in the local women's hospital as part of a specialized program for mothers with a history of substance use that is designed to keep them together with their babies following birth. During that time she had lost her housing at Wenonah House due to prior repeated rule violations. When she left the hospital she was forced to go back to Fern Grove, but this time her daughter was allowed to come with her. Lula told me that she loved being with her baby but that, cut off from Jeff and her friends, she also felt increasingly overcome with anxiety.

I spoke with Lula on the phone only days before she ran away from Fern Grove following a major altercation with program staff. Lula's anxiety had gotten so bad that she had asked to be taken to St. Paul's Hospital. While there she ran into a friend, and the two of them were observed going into the hospital bathroom at the same time. The staff member who accompanied Lula to the hospital became suspicious that she may have used or picked up drugs while in the bathroom and upon returning to Fern Grove insisted on a full body search. They found some used syringes in the bottom of her backpack and a flap of fentanyl in her wallet. Lula insisted that these items had been left there by Jeff a long time ago. Rather than wait to get kicked out—although it was not clear to me from her retelling whether that was the course of action that the program staff intended to take—Lula chose to abruptly leave Fern Grove, telling them that she was "not in the right state of mind to look after her daughter." Lula viewed this as a responsible decision, but from what I could piece together it was primarily the fact that she had abandoned her daughter and left Fern Grove that ultimately resulted in the removal of her child from her custody (although the items found on her after the trip to St. Paul's would not have helped). Lula found herself homeless for the first time since 2012 and quickly relapsed on meth. She began staying at a series of shelters and occasionally crashing with Jeff at the Greystone Hotel. By the time the two of them were sitting in the office that day in late 2017, it was clear that they were once again together.

Lula was devastated by the loss of custody of her daughter, and I was very worried about her. She had told me over the phone that she felt like she had worked hard at Fern Grove, only to be accused of using drugs and told that she wasn't good enough to be a mom to her daughter—an assessment that she vehemently disagreed with. She said there were many moments since leaving Fern Grove when she thought about killing herself. "Once again, I'm getting absolutely nowhere, no matter how hard I try," she told me through choking sobs.

I was also worried about Jeff, whose fentanyl use continued to escalate. I knew that he had experienced at least one overdose that year that had required hospitalization. Jeff had long ago stopped taking methadone because he hated the way that it dulled his high and his senses. He told me once that methadone made him feel "zombie-ish" and he felt physically and mentally healthier without it. In general Jeff had told me many times that he had no interest in treatment; without drugs, he was miserable. "Drugs aren't my problem," he insisted. "I would say, if anything, that *lack* of drugs is the problem."

I felt at a loss as to how to help Lula and Jeff, even as I knew that was not a role I could often play in the lives of those I followed. Lula talked vaguely about how she was going to get her daughter back, but she seemed to have no fight left in her. Jeff sat there in pointed silence, making it clear that was not a plan he foresaw coming to fruition nor one he planned to support. I wanted to know where Lula was living and when we might see each other next (possibly without Jeff), but on that day Lula refused to make these kinds of plans with me. I asked her if she wanted any kind of support that I could help to facilitate.

"I'm not interested in treatment or any of that," she replied curtly, as she gathered up her jacket, backpack, and the battered phone she had been charging and prepared to leave. Then she added, almost casually, "As I see it, it's basically your job now to witness my death." Without skipping a beat, she continued, "Just promise me one thing. *Promise me* that you'll look into the circumstances if I do die. I *might not overdose*, right? And I don't want to be added into those numbers if it's not true. Especially, because, like, I'm Native, and there is this whole thing where people are talking about like, a lot of Native people dying from overdoses right now. I sure as *hell* don't want to die down here as one of their statistics." She stormed out of the office.

Over the years I have played the moment when Lula said this to me over and over in my mind. Even now I can hardly bear to write and read those words back, and yet they also continue to strike me as incredibly important. In this moment it seems to me that Lula expressed multiple refusals: refusals to go to/ on treatment, to submit to the gaze of research, and to be (mis)recognized as "just another" Indigenous youth overdose death (Coulthard 2014; Simpson 2014). Like the Inuit youth described by Lisa Stevenson (2014) who were (and are still) contending with the suicide epidemic in Canada's North, Indigenous young people in Vancouver are being asked to cooperate in their own survival by going to residential treatment, taking lifesaving pharmacotherapies like Suboxone, and submitting to various forms of surveillance. But Lula and some of the other Indigenous young people I knew, such as Raymond and Aaron, generally refused to be drawn into this relationship of cooperation with the care assemblage, even as culturally safe youth-focused treatment programs are made increasingly available. Lula, Raymond, and Aaron all had a long history of being drawn into the churn of state-sponsored intervention. Experiences of government care, incarceration, and hospitalization across their own young lives and inter-generational experiences of institutionalization informed a felt knowledge of the broken promises and forms of stagnation, violence, and loss that can result. From the Indian Act to Canada's recent endorsement of the United Nations Declaration on the Rights of Indigenous People, the colonial past and present is rife with promises of a different, better future offered in return for particular kinds of cooperation. These promises are often violently and abruptly broken. In this context the sense of future promise that can be generated by intervention may not only ring false but even signal danger and disaster, such as the loss of child custody. Lula, Raymond, and Aaron were perhaps not so much falling through the cracks as following different lines of potential in a land of broken promises powerfully shaped by history. This broken promise land was also shaped by the postwelfare neoliberal state, in which opportunities to attain various markers of the good life—housing, employment, leisure, upward mobility—are rapidly dissolving for those at the bottom of socioeconomic hierarchies.

THE BROKEN PROMISE LAND

Accelerating intervention across youth-focused treatment settings continues to be fueled by a desperate desire to *do something* to stem the tide of deaths locally. Of course no one whose job it is to address the overdose public health emergency intends to hold out treatment as a promise of a bright and shiny future. If, as Bharat Venkat (2016) has argued, treatment constitutes a promise of sorts, it is one that is frequently broken by the near inevitability of relapse. What is less well understood, perhaps, is that among many young people the broken promises of treatment do not necessarily lie in the limitations of particular programs and pharmacotherapies or even in the numerous "gaps" generated by a fragmented system of mental health and addictions care (Government of BC 2019). Rather, they are located in history and the postwelfare neoliberal state and registered affectively as a crushing sense of stagnation or endless stops and starts ("Things are not going to get any better," "I can't get anywhere").

Low treatment access and retention rates among young people cannot be explained just by pointing to gaps and barriers in systems of care for adolescents and young adults (Dreifuss et al. 2013; Schuman-Olivier et al. 2014; Vo et al. 2016; Winters et al. 2014). We also need to reckon with the kind of selective bio-politics at work in settings like Vancouver, where treatment can perhaps improve young people's chances of accessing various poverty management and public health services, but nevertheless often still leaves them living in undesirable housing, barely scraping by on a crap job or meager monthly welfare payments, firmly locked out of their dreams of place in the city.

"I don't make promises to youth about housing and jobs and stuff like that anymore," one manager at a residential program told me with real anguish in her voice. "There have been times in the past when it seemed easier to find them a place to live, and we could work on those things together. But not now. And it's really heartbreaking not to be able to offer them something, especially when they are doing *everything* we are asking of them and not putting a single foot wrong in terms of the plan we have developed for them. But at the same time we need to prepare them for the reality of what's out there."

Or what's not out there. The city and province acknowledge the importance of housing, employment, income, and tackling structural and historical forms of inequality and oppression in order to address the current overdose crisis and fix the system of mental health and addictions care. However, change in these areas was coming far too slowly for many of those I knew. Even as access to evidence-based treatment and care increased dramatically, this did not necessarily constitute a "pathway to hope" (to use the title of a 2019 report that provides a roadmap for remaking the provincial mental health and addictions system; Government of BC 2019). Rather, many young people had a deeply troubling sense that they were getting lost or going nowhere within a system of services that still could not help them achieve any semblance of the futures they were longing for. Alarmingly, for some the churn of intervention across youth-focused services could actually seem to exacerbate harm when individuals were repeatedly caught up in a sense of momentum and promise only to be faced with a rapid descent into stagnation when their plans for the future fell through, stalled, and dead-ended.

In this context many young people expressed a commitment to the thing that could be counted on to propel them forward in the present: the frenetic fun of intensive meth and fentanyl use.[22] As Aaron Goodfellow (2008) reminds us, it is easy to translate individuals' drug use beyond the grasp of lifesaving programs into institutionally authorized forms. Their evasions and refusals of treatment and housing programs and even harm reduction thereby become a reflection of pathology, symptoms of untreated substance use and concurrent psychiatric disorders, or gaps and barriers to access. This framing further fuels the will to intervene. Anthropologists, alternatively, might read young people's evasions and refusals through the lens of resistance.[23] I, however, am focused on something else: affect's potential to engender deep ambivalence toward treatment and other interventions in the context of successive waves of public health emergency, which sometimes crystalized into moments of withdrawal, evasion, and refusal.

JANET, JOHNNY, RACHEL, AND GORDO, CAMP UNDER THE TRACKS, 2017

By 2017 Janet had been living in various suburbs of Greater Vancouver for seven years. She was one of the few young people I had followed since 2008 who completely avoided living in supportive housing buildings downtown. She told me on several occasions that she preferred to have her freedom, camping on the edges of construction sites and in semiforested areas with a series of boyfriends and squatting in empty homes or renting rooms in run-down houses when they got tired of sleeping outside. At least once or twice a year Janet would move indoors while her boyfriends were in jail, couch surfing with friends, ex-boyfriends, and those she referred to as sugar daddies. Janet once attributed her ability to live under these widely varied conditions to excelling in Girl Scouts and Cadet training as a child.

Janet had gone to detox at least once in 2010 while she was still living downtown. But from 2010 to 2017 I never heard her talk about detox or treatment, although she did regularly talk to me about how she moderated her substance use by fine-tuning combinations of licit and illicit substances to mediate withdrawal symptoms and cravings and help her sleep. Back when she had been using heroin and crack daily, it was "shitloads of meth" that eventually allowed her to stop the former (Fast et al. 2014). Since she had started using meth intensively, it was a combination of energy drinks, coffee, cannabis, and alcohol that allowed her to slow down or take breaks when she needed to (Paul et al. 2020). When her alcohol use started to get too intense she switched back to doing more meth in order to "sober up."

Unlike some of those I knew, Janet didn't seem to be evading Vancouver's care assemblage because of repeated past negative experiences with "the system," although she also spent much of her adolescence cycling between government group homes and juvenile detention. Instead, she reflected that when she was growing up—as now—she was simply unable to live harmoniously with most other people or according to someone else's rules. She had been able to live in the old SROs for some time back when they were largely lawless; however, as soon as those SROs began being converted into supportive housing, she knew it was time to leave. Janet also told me on more than one occasion that supportive housing and "all those other services" didn't give you the "push" you needed to make something of yourself and your life. They didn't really help you to finish school or some kind of training or to get a job. Instead, they trapped you downtown and "got you nowhere."

Throughout 2017 I visited Janet at the camp she shared with her longtime on-again, off-again boyfriend Johnny. We always met each other at a nearby SkyTrain station before heading off along a busy roadway in the direction of the intersection where Janet and a number of others squeegeed and used drugs each day. As soon as we had greeted each other at the entrance to the station, Janet always immediately launched into an elaborate story about the latest drama between her and Johnny. The roar of nearby traffic and rapid pace of her speech made it difficult for me to follow what she was saying, and I always had to ask her to repeat herself once we were at her camp. This also allowed me to record many of our conversations at the camp.

In 2017 Janet and Johnny were sharing their Port Coquitlam camp with twenty-year-old Rachel and nineteen-year-old Gordo. At the intersection where they all squeegeed, Gordo could almost always be seen picking his way back and forth along a narrow concrete island in the middle of the road, attempting to solicit customers stopped at the traffic light. He approached each driver-side window, lifting his dripping squeegee into the air in a questioning—if also somewhat intimidating—gesture. When there were no takers, he would often make the split-second decision to wash one of the windshields anyways, with the hope that the driver would feel compelled to roll down the window and push some spare change into his hand. As the light turned green and he sometimes lost his chance to collect any money, he would slam down his gear and begin swearing and gesturing wildly, teetering precariously as the traffic sped past. Other times someone would give him money regardless of whether he had washed their windshield. This both pleased and infuriated him and the handful of others who worked on that corner, most of whom preferred to feel like they were working for a living and not just accepting charity. And yet many including Janet also panhandled at the gas station on the northwest corner of the intersection.

As we arrived at the intersection one particularly sweltering day in summer 2017 Janet yelled at Gordo to "chill the f-ck out," explaining to me that his erratic behavior was what sometimes got them kicked off the intersection by local police. Since I had last seen her a couple of months prior Janet's hair had grown out into a shaggy bob and she had dyed it bright red. She looked sporty in hightop sneakers, yoga pants, and a tube top pulled up over a sports bra. Rachel was sitting cross-legged on the sidewalk, nodding off against a post. Her scruffy Pomeranian was curled up in her lap. Although the two of them were in a patch of shade created by the SkyTrain tracks that loomed overhead, the dog looked miserable. Janet scooped him up and took him to the gas station across the street, where she wet him down and refilled his water bowl. I placed the large double cream, double sugar coffee I had brought Rachel from Tim Hortons a short distance away from where she was sitting and waved at Gordo to get his attention so that he would know I had brought something for him too.

At that time both Rachel and Gordo were using meth daily and fentanyl regularly. Rachel told me that the fentanyl allowed her to come down and sleep after several daylong binges on meth. It also relieved her anxiety and pain: physical, emotional, and psychological. The meth, on the other hand, got her going: it dissolved the crushing weight of the depression that she had been managing since she was a child and gave her the energy she needed to squeegee each day or occasionally engage in sex work (Fast et al. 2014). Janet and Johnny also regularly described their meth use in these kinds of utilitarian terms. But Gordo and Rachel were also always careful to tell me that using drugs was very, very fun. Like Janet and Johnny, Rachel and Gordo said that they had no interest in accessing treatment or any other kinds of services. One reason that they liked living out in the suburbs was that, other than a single outreach van that provided them with harm reduction supplies, they were largely "left alone." This was a stark contrast to downtown Vancouver, where it was much more difficult—though not impossible, they all agreed—to evade various workers.

After an hour or so Janet and I left the intersection, following a wide gravel path that took us along a highway embankment, its yellowed grass baking in the sun. We passed a few other small camps that were reasonably well camouflaged by the dense foliage on the opposite side of the path. Evidence of their existence was sparse during the daytime anyways: a string tied between two trees overlaid with cardboard to provide shade, a mattress covered with a tarp weighed down by several rocks. Janet told me that the police generally allowed people to inhabit these places provided that any garbage was cleared out daily and that most possessions were packed up and hidden during the daytime. During a previous visit she had shown me where she used to hide her stuff when she first moved out here. A short distance away from the highway there was a small bridge. On the underside of each end of the bridge was a sort of concrete shelf several meters deep but only a meter or so high, which could be reached by scrambling up a steep concrete embankment. Tents, tarps, pillows, and squeegee gear were pushed up against the far end of the shelf and hung up on some piping along the underside of the bridge. Janet told me that she had also slept there for a few weeks when she first arrived in the area and still occasionally did so when she and Johnny had a particularly bad fight.

As we continued toward her camp Janet kept up a steady stream of dialogue about what she and Johnny had been fighting about. Janet was angry that Johnny was undertaking highly risky breaking and entering jobs, meaning that it was just a matter of time before he was caught and sent back to jail for another couple of months. The two of them still occasionally took on "legitimate" landscaping jobs, but the business that they had been running with some success a few years earlier had largely fallen apart when Johnny started cycling in and out of jail and his truck was impounded. Meanwhile, Johnny was angry that Janet was squeegeeing and occasionally panhandling outside the gas station, which he viewed as beneath them. Janet told me that despite being in and out of jail and homeless for the previous five years, Johnny was still holding onto the idea that they had a "perfect life"—or that a perfect life was just around the corner. Janet was increasingly desperate and impatient for that life to begin too. She wanted her and Johnny to find work, move into a place together, and finally get married. Meanwhile, Johnny was still not divorced from his wife, and Janet saw nothing wrong with squeegeeing and panhandling to make the money she needed for smokes, junk food, and alcohol. Janet told me that Johnny was responsible for bringing in the money for their meth use, although I noticed she had no problem getting some when he absconded for days at a time, which happened frequently. During these periods they both developed intense jealousies regarding whom the other was with and what the other was doing. The drama between them was fueled by the rumors and gossip that circulated rapidly among those in their networks, which fanned out across the suburbs of Port Coquitlam, Burnaby, and New Westminster and included ex-romantic partners and friend-dealer-users who were happy to escalate the strife between them. Janet admitted that the previous day Johnny had flown into a rage and packed up all of her stuff, telling her to get lost. He had also punched her in the face, leaving a reddish-purple bruise over one of her eyes. Not for the first time, I asked her why she stayed with Johnny, when she was so clearly able to take care of herself. The answer changed each time I asked:

"He makes a bit more money than me."
"It's easier out here with someone."
"I love the shit out of him. I really do."

When we finally arrived at her camp I noticed that her stuff was back inside their tent—evidence, perhaps, that the worst of the fight with Johnny was over. In fact, everything looked immaculate, as usual. I had spent many hours watching Janet meticulously arrange and re-arrange her things, whether she was living out of a backpack, at a camp, or in a rented room. She often joked that she was OCD about keeping things tidy, organized, and clean. This kind of obsessive tinkering with things is also a common effect of meth use.

The camp that Janet, Johnny, Rachel, and Gordo shared was far enough away from everything that the police allowed them to keep their tents and other stuff set up during the day. This allowed both tents to be furnished with carpeting, mattresses, decorative stuffed toys, and candles. Janet and Johnny's tent even had a chair in one corner. There was running water nearby, and the four of them had fashioned a dish-washing area at the base of one of the concrete legs of the SkyTrain tracks that ran directly overhead. Between the two tents were a few mismatched lawn chairs, a highly unsteady plastic table with three good remaining legs, and a rusty and disused grill.

Janet sank down angrily into one of the faded mesh chairs and began furiously texting Johnny, who she was suddenly certain was off at a friend-dealer-user's house doing meth instead of selling the things he had stolen earlier in the day. While she was constantly anxious about the possibility of Johnny being sent back to jail, Janet was also adamant that he should be out there making money. She wanted that income to come from landscaping, painting, or construction work, which she believed Johnny could easily acquire if only he would apply himself. But it seemed to me that he had been almost exclusively resorting to breaking and entering since his truck was impounded several years prior. It also seemed to me that it was Janet who still clung tightly to dreams of growing a landscaping business with Johnny or moving to Fort McMurray together to do highly lucrative construction work, whereas Johnny viewed those dreams as increasingly out of reach. His disillusionment was one reason why he often flew into rages when he saw Janet squeegeeing on the corner and panhandling in front of the gas station or when he returned to their camp, no matter how immaculately tidied it was.

Finally, over an hour later Johnny texted Janet back to say that he was on his way. While we were waiting Janet and I picked some blackberries from the huge bushes that lined the gravel path leading to their camp. We had been at it for forty-five minutes when we finally saw Johnny coming down the path. He was walking his BMX bike, a pizza box balanced on the handlebars. Gordo and Rachel were with him. Johnny was much later than he said he would be, and I could almost feel Janet's temper rising as she stood beside me holding a plastic yogurt container full of blackberries. I braced myself for an altercation, but once we were all standing together Johnny and Janet both just offered each other the food they had procured without saying much else. That wordless peace offering seemed to be enough to make it clear that Johnny had scored meth for her, and the two of them took off quickly in the direction of the camp so that Janet could use.

Rachel, Gordo, and I ambled back to the camp at a much slower pace, their tiny dog following behind us. The couple was in a talkative and generous mood, asking me all sorts of questions about my research and if I would like to meet so-and-so and so-and-so out here so that I could get a better sense of things. We arrived to find Janet and Johnny still in their tent, murmuring quietly to one another. Gordo pulled his own recently acquired BMX out of his tent and began fiddling with the pedals and gears, providing a somewhat difficult-to-follow description of the modifications he planned to make to the bike. Rachel sat with me on the lawn chairs and asked me bluntly, "So what do you want—or, to know—from us?"

"I'm not totally sure," I admitted carefully. I knew Rachel's patience with me and my questions had its limits. Her generous mood could change quickly to one of annoyance or even anger. "My research right now is really focused on the overdose crisis and responses to it, like treatment," I began. "But I know you guys have said a few times to me that that is not something you are interested in—"

"Well, I *did* actually go to treatment when I was seventeen," Rachel interrupted me. She stood up suddenly and began pacing back and forth in front of her tent, obsessively adjusting and readjusting the pink wig she was wearing with one hand and managing not to spill the last dregs of the coffee I had brought her with the other. I was amazed that she still had the coffee, even though it had been several hours since I had left it for her. "When I was seventeen, I punched a cop in the face and that sent me to treatment. If you get in trouble with the law, you'll get in [to residential treatment] *really* fast. And you know what else I got? I became a youth in [government] care, and I got a bunch of, you know, money and waivers and bursaries for school and stuff. But my thinking was I'm on drugs, this is something I have, this is fun, and what am I giving it up for, anyways? What am I surviving *for*? Oh, you want me to get a crap job? Oh, okay, I'm gonna have to pay this student loan off for the rest of my life and I'm never gonna be able to actually have a *good* job—I'm gonna be one paycheck away from home-lessness my entire life? Oh, *great*."

She looked me straight in the eye and asked provocatively, "What do *you* think about that?"

EXITS, JANET, 2015

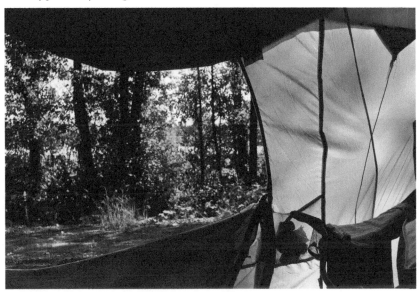

JORDAN, RAIN CITY, 2016

Jordan overdosed and died in his room at the Beachwood Hotel in 2016. He was twenty-seven years old. Shae called to tell me the news and inform me of the small memorial that was being held in a park that Jordan loved in the Downtown Eastside. We stood there in the spitting rain, huddled under umbrellas. A few people shared stories and memories. There was hushed and not-so-hushed conversation about how many people were now dying in the way that Jordan had. Across the Rain City cherry blossoms began to explode in delicate profusions of pink.[1] Two weeks later the overdose public health emergency was declared by the provincial government.

LAURA, FIELD OFFICE, 2017

Laura came into the field office in the spring of 2017 and said that she wanted to participate in the new treatment study I was running. We sat down in the office that day and ended up talking for almost two hours. I got the sense that Laura was well practiced at these kinds of encounters; she seemed to know how to make herself comfortable in the hard chair, alternating between sitting cross-legged and pulling her knees up against her chest, her chin resting on her delicate, clasped hands. Laura was twenty-two years old and very pretty. She was carefully made up with heavy black eyeliner, dark lipstick, and long, straightened brown hair dyed red at the tips. She wore a baggy monochrome white sweat suit and colorful high-top sneakers.

Laura said that she had been in and out of the psychiatric ward, residential drug treatment, shelters, and supportive housing since she was sixteen. She had long struggled with an eating disorder, anxiety, and depression and had started using alcohol, meth, and heroin intensively in her teens. Most recently she had attended Fern Grove during the early stages of a pregnancy that ended in a miscarriage. Laura was certain it was the antipsychotic medication that she had been forced to take through an Extended Leave agreement that had caused the miscarriage. She described to me how she had gradually and painstakingly convinced her doctors to take her off the medication, but not in time to change the outcome of her pregnancy.

Laura was very in love with her boyfriend. Like so many others, they had both hoped the pregnancy and having a child together would catalyze dramatic changes in their lives, but it had not worked out that way. Instead, Laura's time at Fern Grove had only further confirmed her sense that stays in residential treatment and the psychiatric ward got her "absolutely nowhere."

She reflected, "I feel like I go into those places and it's always the same thing. Like when I go to the psych ward, right, they just put me on medications and tell me to rest and watch TV. I just sit around and wait and *nothing* happens— nobody does anything. And I'll even be like, 'Is there anything else I can do?' Because I still, like, have a lot of goals for myself. 'Why don't you guys help me?' And they're like, 'Well, you're just here to rest and gain a couple pounds.' And then eventually they rush me out and I'm back on the street."

Laura acknowledged that her time at Fern Grove, and at a different, youth-dedicated residential treatment center that she had also attended during the previous year, could have been much more helpful than her time in the psychiatric ward. She said that she particularly liked learning about the science of addiction during group sessions. But at both Fern Grove and the treatment center her antipsychotic medication had made it impossible to fully participate. "I was just really, really tired the whole time," she said. "If I had not been on the [antipsychotic] shot I would have benefited so much more because I wouldn't have been so zonked out. But on the shot you can't really do anything. You can't get out of bed. You don't feel happiness from all of the activities."

Laura had recently concluded that the best way to work on her goals was to do it on her own. She told me that her biggest priority was avoiding being put back on an antipsychotic injection because if that happened it would be much harder to stay off meth. When she was on the antipsychotic, she needed meth to wake herself up and get going. She got caught in a loop, in which she was forced to take an antipsychotic injection because of her intensive meth use and the risk of psychosis, and she continued to use meth because of the sedating effects of the antipsychotic.

Laura said that to avoid being put back on an antipsychotic she needed to attend all of her appointments at YouthNow and demonstrate during those appointments that she was off drugs, adequately managing her mental health, and working toward her goals. She described how she carefully curated her performance at these appointments to give the impression that everything was going well.

"Literally, at the last appointment, I was like, I gotta look like I'm *not* anxious. I gotta look like I'm *not* depressed. I gotta look like I have everything under control." She laughed shakily. "I'm gonna get a job. I'm not relapsing. Everything is good. Everything is good." She paused. "And I actually somehow pulled it off and the psychiatrist didn't threaten to put me back on the antipsychotic! But she's just, like, waiting for me to relapse. You know, 'Relapse is a part of recovery' and 'We're here for you if you do relapse' and all that stuff that they say that I really don't want to hear, right? Like, I don't want to be a drug addict for the rest of my life."

To a certain extent, things were going well for Laura. She and her boyfriend were no longer living in supportive housing downtown. Instead, they were crashing in her boyfriend's parents' basement, trying to support each other with staying off meth and fentanyl. Laura had been off meth for several weeks and was seeing improvements in her mental health. But she admitted that she and her boyfriend had been using opioids at least once a week. She didn't want to tell her care providers at YouthNow about this, though, in case they could somehow use it as an excuse to put her back on the antipsychotic.

A few days after our first conversation Laura came into the field office again. She said that she found it motivating to come to the office to participate in the study. It was "really keeping her going" with the changes that she was trying to make in her life. We had another long, detailed conversation about her experiences moving in and out of treatment and the life that she and her boyfriend wanted to create together. She said that they planned to get married in the next couple of years. She talked about wanting to attend a meditation retreat to help her with the more spiritual aspects of her recovery.

Two weeks later, I went down to the field office to listen to a voicemail from Laura's mom, informing me that Laura had died from an overdose just one week after our second conversation. Her mom asked if I would be willing to call her and possibly meet for coffee. In the days before her death Laura had talked about me and the study a few times. She had seemed happy and motivated. Could I help her to make sense of what had happened? I said that I couldn't share the details of my conversations with Laura but agreed to meet. We sat in a coffee shop and talked for a long time about Laura, how well she had seemed to be doing, and whether it was possible that something other than an overdose had taken her life. Could the doctors have been wrong about what had happened? It seemed to Laura's mom, as it had to Laura herself, that the many doctors Laura had seen had so often been wrong about what she needed across her young life.

SHAE/TRIX, APARTMENT, 2017

At the end of 2014 Shae secured a rent subsidy via a new BC Housing program designed to stabilize individuals with mental health issues who were at risk of homelessness in market rental housing. In 2014, Shae did not seem to identify with either of these descriptors; during that year whenever we spoke, they were far more preoccupied with their physical rather than mental health and had not experienced street-based homelessness in years, except when they were choosing to sleep outside rather than return to their room at Arbutus House. But as they prepared for an interview to determine their eligibility for the new program, Shae told me they had recently noticed that anyone who used drugs to "keep themselves alive" in downtown Vancouver now seemed to be classified as "having a mental health problem." Performing the twinning of mental health and addictions during the eligibility interview was their way out of Arbutus House. During the interview Shae would have to walk a fine line between demonstrating that they needed housing and mental health support from the nonprofit that was delivering the program, but not so much support that they should remain in Arbutus House.

Across the years I knew Shae they had always been a smooth talker and very charming. I was not surprised, therefore, when they messaged me to say that they had been approved for the program. Shae was assigned an outreach worker from the nonprofit who helped them to secure a one-bedroom, ground-floor apartment on a quiet residential street in Burnaby. From there, the goal was stability. Over the next several years Shae would receive regular visits from the outreach worker to help them navigate the transition from supportive to market rental housing and build the kinds of life skills (e.g., cleaning, cooking, budgeting, liaising with a landlord) that would allow them to remain in market rental housing in the future.

The squat, three-story building that Shae moved into in January 2015 sat across from an old church, beyond which it was possible to see the tips of the North Shore Mountains. The apartment building was old but well maintained. The lawn out front was neatly mowed, and rows of clipped coniferous hedges concealed the ground-floor patios—one of which now belonged to Shae. The first time I visited them at their apartment just shortly after they had moved in, Shae greeted me from this prized patio, waving from behind the hedges and smiling widely.

Inside the building the fluorescent-lit hallways were narrow and dingy and smelled strongly of stale cigarette smoke. But as I entered Shae's apartment for the first time I saw that it was spacious, with lots of natural sunlight. It was Sunday, and when I arrived Shae was in the middle of cleaning. That was what they did now on Sundays, they told me proudly, although they had been there only a few short weeks. In a galley-style kitchen decorated with faded flower print tiles, the dishes were done and stacked neatly on a tea towel to dry. The bathroom had been freshly mopped and smelled of disinfectant. A sea of toiletries was meticulously arranged on the counter. The living room and bedroom were still a mess, every surface piled high with discarded clothes, makeup, papers, and multiple ash trays full of cigarette butts. I knew from Facebook that Shae had been doing a lot of drag shows. Two of Trix's dresses hung in one of the windows of the living room, and her wigs and shoes took up most of a large bookshelf. In the midst of various detritus on the living room table was a poinsettia plant, the vibrant red flowers emerging from shiny gold cellophane wrapping. It must have been left over from the holidays. Judging by the food bowl on the floor by the entrance to the kitchen, Shae had a cat.

They told me that everything felt lighter now that they were living in a normal home. The deck and its clipped hedges, the kitchen with its flower print tiles, cleaning on Sundays, a cat—these were some of the things, perhaps, that constituted so many young people's dreams of place in Vancouver. And then there was what had been subtracted. "Here I don't have staff check on me. I don't need to sign in my guests," Shae listed. "They can buzz me and I can buzz them in—I don't need to go down and get them. They don't need to leave ID." The lightness they described was apparent in their tone of voice and demeanor, even their dress. While we talked Shae sprawled on the floor by the sliding glass doors of the balcony, wearing jeans and a T-shirt despite the cold weather, chain-smoking cigarettes. They were so much less fidgety than usual.

"I feel like a whole new person here, right? I'm *so* much happier," Shae gushed at one point. "People have even said that I'm *calmer*. And I've put weight on!" Shae told me they had barely used meth since moving and were doing less sex work. Dates used to be their way out of downtown, across bridges and viaducts and away into adjacent neighborhoods and suburbs. Now, one of those routes out was their way home.

Later in the conversation Shae admitted, "I still feel a little on edge—just edgy. Living here is just, like, so different from what I've been used to, right? But I'm just slowing walking around the neighborhood, trying to get to know Burnaby. It's much more—quieter. Here. But I think I can get used to it."

I visited Shae regularly at their apartment throughout 2015 and 2016. One year into living there Shae was still grateful not to be living in supportive housing, still doing lots of drag shows, and still mostly not using meth. They also still seemed to be somewhat on edge, as though they were balancing precariously between settling into their new life and letting their old life go.

"I told my outreach worker, this is *make or break* for me, being out here," Shae reflected on one occasion. It was February 2016, and we were sitting together on their balcony enjoying the late afternoon sun that was rare for Vancouver during that time of year. "I'm in my late-ish twenties now, right? And if I can't, like, find a way to, like, make some form of a life out here, then I am going to end my [rent] subsidy and go to the Downtown Eastside and let my life go. And there have been moments, lately, when I've really thought about, like, doing that—for some reason."

Shae tried to make sense of what was driving them back downtown. They pondered whether their "addict's mentality" was to blame or something else they couldn't quite put their finger on. Shae admitted that they were bored. Although at one point they had managed to strike up a complicated friendship with an older woman who lived one floor above them, Shae felt isolated and alone much of the time.

"Living out here has been a blessing but I miss the chaos, I miss the stress, I miss the drama, I miss being needed by people," Shae said toward the end of that conversation in 2016. "It's a comfort thing, right? That life [downtown] is the only thing I'm comfortable with, after so many years. I feel like I'm not really *doing* anything out here, most days. I've been here for a year and what do I really have to, like, show for it?" They continued quickly, "But I've been looking into this, um, organic, like medication—it comes from a root, from some place in, uh, Africa? It resets your whole—everything in your mind, so that you go back to how you were pre-using drugs. And like, in a week of using that, like, you should be back to—like, as if you never had an addiction. So I've been thinking *that's* what I might need, right?"

The last time I visited Shae at their apartment in the summer of 2017 they greeted me as Trix. I was barely through the front door when they told me that they were thinking about transitioning and might want to be called Trix rather than Shae. I asked Trix which pronouns they identified with, wanting to adjust my thinking and language as quickly as possible. But the answer was still forming, perhaps. Trix told me they identified as both a boy and a girl and that none of the available pronouns were exactly right. They weren't totally sure if they wanted to give up the name Shae entirely.

The apartment was messier than I had ever seen it. There was a mattress in the middle of the living room covered with an accumulation of miscellaneous stuff. A large mirror was propped up against a living room table beside the mattress. Trix told me that they were having more regulars (sex work dates) over these days. They had a new boyfriend who loved the ambiguity of their gender identity, although he was still in the closet.

Trix said that their mom had recently died in an accident. They seemed to be both devastated and emboldened by this loss. Trix's mom could never accept their sexuality, gender identity, and HIV status. It was their mom's death, Trix said, that had released something in them so that they could start thinking about transitioning. But it had also pulled them down into another period of depression that was deepened when their close friend, Tom, died from an overdose in his SRO room downtown. In the months and days leading up to his death, Tom had been crashing at Trix's apartment regularly. Trix said that they still could not sit on the couch where Tom had slept night after night, even though it was now many months later.

"I'm still kind of lost from what happened," Trix said shakily, picking at their bare nails. They told me that after the death of their mom and friend they had started using heroin/fentanyl again. Initially, it had been a way to balance out their increasing meth use. Then, it had become a way to sink down further into grief and loss. "With losing my mom and then Tom, it just seemed like I hit rock bottom," Trix said. "And then, like, I almost wanted to stay in that depression mode."

It struck me that Trix had not yet been able to settle into the new life that they had envisioned when they first got their apartment in the suburbs. They continued to feel lost in the city in many moments, a sense of being unmoored that was intensified by the loss of their mom, Tom, and many others. Trix continued to be driven back downtown, to the Never Never Land of the drug scenes there, where they and so many other young people had made new, complicated families with each other. These already fragile families were increasingly buffeted and battered by public health emergencies—which by 2020 included the COVID-19 pandemic—and a steady churn of intervention that oftentimes unintentionally increased isolation. Yet they persisted. It was still possible to go back downtown and sense being at the center of something rife with potential. It was downtown that Trix met their new boyfriend. And it was this new boyfriend, and thinking about transitioning, that seemed to be a way back up to the surface of the life Trix desired. They told me that they had been using less heroin/fentanyl and meth since they started to seriously consider taking hormones. They had even recently entered a contest at IKEA for a before-and-after transformation of their apartment.

"I still live in boxes here—like, I'm still in boxes, right?" Trix gestured around the living room with a hand that was now manicured with bright pink stick-on nails, except for one missing pinky nail that we had not been able to find anywhere. "I'm not fully unpacked in the ways that I want to be, because I don't have things. And I don't—like, I don't know how to, like, set up my place to make it a *home*."

Each time I visited Trix I noticed that there continued to be several large blue Rubbermaid tubs piled in their bedroom and living room, so evocative of where they had come from. I had seen these exact same plastic tubs in the supportive housing rooms of so many young people over the years. It was a way to protect those possessions they were able to hold onto across multiple moves between shelters, SROs, supportive housing sites, and treatment and recovery houses. Until Trix unpacked and got rid of those tubs they might never feel truly settled. But if they let go of those tubs they were also perhaps letting go of a form of life that Trix was not confident they were done with.

JANET, RECOVERY HOUSE, 2018

In mid-2018, Janet started talking in earnest about moving indoors. She told me that she didn't want to spend another winter outside. However, I got the sense that her desire to move in somewhere with Johnny had more to do with solidifying their commitment to each other than with her inability to continue camping. Johnny was still not divorced from his wife and continued to regularly take off from their camp in Port Coquitlam for long periods of time. Janet had caught him cheating on her a number of times and regularly called and texted me to tell me how unhappy she was.

Yet she continued to try to make things work between them. In a sort of half-hearted compromise, they began squatting in a series of empty houses instead of camping. Then they moved into a recovery house so that Johnny might meet the conditions of, and eventually get off, probation. Staying at the recovery house gave him a fixed address where he could meet his curfew each night. It ostensibly demonstrated that he was "working a [Twelve Step] program" and "trying to stay out of trouble." However, the reality was that Johnny was dealing meth to recovery house residents, most of whom were actively using. This included Janet for the first two months they were there. And then she abruptly stopped using and began eagerly embracing the daily routines that were tentatively in place despite the active drug use that was also occurring. These routines included waking up each morning at seven thirty, attending several Twelve Step meetings each week, daily journaling and Twelve Step work, and keeping up with various chores.

On a blustery afternoon in November I took the SkyTrain out to Surrey to visit Janet at the recovery house. At this point she and Johnny had been living there for three months. We had planned that Janet would meet me at the bus loop adjacent to the SkyTrain station and we would travel together to the house, but at the last minute she called to say that I would need to take the bus by myself. She explained that she was back on "conditions," meaning that she was allowed to leave the house only with two other residents, or "three strong" in recovery house lingo. The previous week the house manager had caught Janet sneaking in the back door after curfew. Janet had insisted the incident was entirely innocent—she was hopped up on energy drinks and had lost track of the time. However, the house manager thought that she was high on meth and kicked her out for several days (during which Johnny snuck her back in each night to sleep). Janet was eventually allowed back into the house but was put on conditions, as she had been when she first arrived.

The recovery house was a classic "Vancouver special": large and boxy and finished with brick and stucco, with a low-pitched roof, small balcony in the front, fenced-in front yard, and large sun deck in the back. When I arrived, Janet answered the door. I removed my shoes and walked with her up thickly carpeted stairs, emerging into a darkened, cavernous living room. A TV flickered in one corner, and as my eyes adjusted I saw two girls sprawled out on couches. They introduced themselves to me, one referring to herself as the newbie. Janet told me that ten of them were staying there in total. For the most part they all got along. They kept as many lights in the house turned off as possible to keep the electricity bill down, although Janet insisted that the house manager made good money from running "this little operation."

In the kitchen the lights were on, and as we entered I saw that Janet had gained some weight. She looked healthy and rested. Janet resumed making herself a smoothie. On a counter opposite from where she had the Magic Bullet whirring sat several bags of unopened perogies and a cutting board crowded with pieces of thickly sliced sausage. Dinner prep was underway. Through the kitchen window I could see several guys huddled together on the back deck, smoking. Johnny was among them. He nodded at me but didn't come in to say hello.

"I'm thirty days clean," Janet whispered excitedly to me in the kitchen. "And I'm pregnant! About two months along, from what I can tell."

"Wow, congratulations!" I said, also trying to keep my voice low. I wondered if she didn't want Johnny to overhear our conversation. "Does Johnny know?" I asked.

"Yeah," she replied, her expression darkening immediately.

"How does he feel about it?"

"Honestly, he's unsure about it. He's *so-so*. He has other kids that he never sees, right? So." Janet took a long drink of her smoothie. "It's definitely, like, causing some problems in our relationship. Mostly because if I *am* pregnant he's worried that he's going to have to finally smarten up and get his shit together. Divorce his stupid wife, because there's no *way* she's getting half his pension once we have a kid together, right? But instead of getting his shit together, like he's been *promising* me for *ages*, so far he has been taking off all day and night and is probably f-cking *cheating* on me." She sighed heavily, but then seemed to will herself to refocus on the positive. "But I'm actually happy. I'm actually *really* happy about it. I've been pregnant so many times, but I've never managed to keep one going this long. I really hope it sticks. I feel like it will because my boobs are super sore and I'm gaining *shitloads* of weight."

Janet and I headed downstairs to the room that she shared with Johnny. It was a decent size—big enough for a double bed, two bedside tables, and a large dresser—and meticulously tidy. A fuzzy blue housecoat hung on a hook between the bed and the dresser, on top of which was a large lamp, alarm clock, and various toiletries and medicines, including a large bottle of Extra Strength Pepto-Bismol that Janet told me belonged to Johnny. He was always sick these days, she said. I could hear the rhythmic creaking of an old dryer in the room next door. Janet told me that while she found this constant soundtrack annoying, being able to wash and dry clothes was one of the best things about being inside. The other good thing was getting to eat three square meals a day. For the time being Janet also seemed content to at least play along with the recovery program that the house manager lackadaisically enforced. She knew that she needed to make big changes if she was on her way to being a mom.

"Have you been to the doctor?" I asked her, as we continued to discuss her pregnancy.

"I'm *way* too afraid to go to the doctor," Janet replied quickly. This admission surprised me because it was so out of character for her. Janet was someone who generally took charge of situations, no matter how difficult. And I knew that she, like so many others, was looking to this pregnancy to change her life. However, she seemed to be in a state of suspension—between knowing and not knowing whether it was real and would "stick," and between knowing and not knowing whether it would be the thing that finally stabilized her tumultuous relationship with Johnny and the chaotic circumstances of their lives.

"What's scaring you about going to the doctor?" I asked. I was a few months pregnant myself and intimately aware that the list of fears could be long.

Janet explained in her rapid, emphatic speech, "Last week I was spotting a bit, and I thought maybe I was miscarrying again but I didn't because my boobs are still *super* sore. So, I'm *positive* I'm still pregnant. No, what I'm actually really afraid of is that they are going to look inside and they're going to tell me something bad about the baby. I'm just, like, worried I took too many meds and they hurt the baby. I'm on, like, Wellbutrin [an antidepressant] for my anxiety. I've been cutting down my use since I started suspecting I was pregnant—like I'm supposed to be on 150 milligrams of Wellbutrin and I've been taking a quarter of that. But still."

Janet changed the subject slightly. She started talking about how she planned to go to Fern Grove as her pregnancy progressed. But she was already worried about what would happen to Johnny and their relationship because the program was only for birthing parents. Johnny needed to stay at the recovery house; otherwise, he would be in breach of his probationary conditions and sent back to jail. Janet was pretty sure it was only her and her ultimatums that occasionally brought Johnny back to the house as it was. If she left to go to Fern Grove and made all of these big life changes without him, she firmly believed that he would end up in jail and their relationship would disintegrate—this time for good.

Janet said that she still loved Johnny, even though he had utterly disappointed her. "He promised me this year that we'd have our own roof over our heads," she said angrily, pacing around their bedroom. "With our own rules. He'd be back at work and so would I. We were supposed to be functioning and *working* drug addicts this year. That's what it was *supposed* to be. Instead we are in a recovery house because he has to be here."

"Why do you stay with him?" I asked her, as I did almost every time we spoke.

She softened. "At the end of the day I've never had a partner that I actually *wanted* to sit and talk about my problems with, *ever*. Things that happened in my past. He saved my life, actually, by caring about me like that. It means something that he wanted to sit down and listen to and be there with me. You know what I mean?"

Several months later Janet called me to say that she and Johnny were living in a motel that his mom was paying for while Johnny underwent radiation and chemotherapy for cancer. She didn't mention the pregnancy, and I didn't ask.

Janet and Johnny had been kicked out of the recovery house shortly after my visit, when Johnny finally got caught breaching his probationary conditions and Janet punched her arm through a window in reaction. Johnny went to jail for a few weeks, where he learned that he had cancer. During this time Janet returned to Port Coquitlam and found them an empty house to squat in. They stayed there together for a few reasonably happy months once Johnny got out of jail, until he left a burning candle unattended and the house caught fire. Then they were sleeping outside again—and fighting frequently about it—until Johnny's mom stepped in.

Talking to me that day on the phone from their motel room, Janet said that she had not been doing well at all since leaving the recovery house. She was using meth intensively and barely sleeping. She had started using fentanyl occasionally to come down off meth. She said that her health was deteriorating. She was struggling with her hep C and various skin infections and had been in and out of the emergency room. During one of those trips she was told by a doctor that she might have diabetes. Janet had an overdose outside the gas station across from where she continued to squeegee occasionally and had to be resuscitated by paramedics. Her teeth were really bothering her and needed to be fixed. She admitted that it was harder to access care outside downtown Vancouver.

As always, I asked her about whether and how I could help her to see a doctor or a dentist. Was she ready to think about treatment for hep C? Even as she acknowledged that her list of health problems had "almost taken her down a few times during the past month," she easily dismissed my concern and offer of help. She told me simply, "I need to get our lives together before I deal with any of that shit. Get us a real place to stay. Get us back to doing demolition work."

Janet continued to be furious with Johnny because he refused to move in with her, even when she was able to find them various places to stay rent free. Since getting out of jail he had been continuing to regularly take off and stay with other women, refusing to answer Janet's texts or phone calls for days and even weeks at a time. During a brief moment when they had made up she grudgingly agreed to stay at the motel with him, using alcohol to calm herself down so that the two of them could cohabitate reasonably peacefully. They had started going out coppering together for several hours every day to make money for drugs and food, despite Johnny's poor health. "I don't really want us to be doing that," Janet admitted. "Because, like, the cops are pretty much onto us and if we get caught we go to jail. Period. But it's also, like, the only quality time we spend together anymore."

Eventually, in late 2019, Janet did leave Johnny. Or perhaps he left her. The exact details were never made clear to me. Johnny moved into supportive housing in Port Coquitlam, and Janet continued to squat, camp, and crash with friends and sugar daddies in various suburbs. She quickly found a new serious boyfriend who, like Johnny, alternated between saving her life and breaking it apart. Over the next two years she spent periods of time using drugs intensively and periods of time off drugs, but never by entering the treatment system. Eventually, she got bored of squeegeeing and coppering and returned to dealing and occasional sex work. The latter were more stressful, perhaps, in terms of the risks and harms that must be navigated daily, but Janet said she felt much less depressed since making the transition. She relocated back to Vancouver and began spending time downtown again. She said that those who still knew or remembered her were surprised to see her back after so many years. What struck her was that there weren't many people around anymore who fell into either category.

"Out of the thirty or forty youth that were together downtown back ten, twelve years ago—there's maybe ten of us who are still alive," she told me over the phone in the summer of 2020. "Most of them have passed away. And of the ten that are still alive, maybe four of us are actually doing good."

Janet had been one of the ones to survive those first, brutal years of the overdose emergency. I don't think this surprised her. It didn't surprise me. Janet was the toughest person I knew, even as her relationship with Johnny and other boyfriends made her tremendously fragile in many moments. But Janet said to me many times over the years that she had done as well as she had because she had stayed away from downtown Vancouver and outside its poverty management and public health infrastructures. What would happen now that she was back downtown?

Of course Janet had no intention of staying put. She never did. Her dream of moving to Fort McMurray to work construction with Johnny had long ago dissolved in the dramatic ups and downs of their relationship. But her next romantic relationship engendered new dreams of place, this time of taking off to the interior of BC to live in a remote cabin in the woods. And even as this new relationship waxed and waned, the dream persisted. Janet knew that she could continue on alone if she had to. At the end of 2020 she told me, "One day, I swear, I'm just going to take off from here without a word. I'll just up and leave and never come back."

EXITS, JANET, 2018

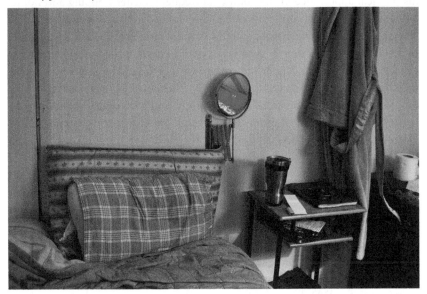

TERRY, PSYCHIATRIC WARD, 2018

In the summer of 2018 Terry sent me a Facebook message to tell me that he was in the psychiatric ward at St. Paul's Hospital. A week earlier he went to the emergency room in a state of extreme agitation about multiple health ailments, including the stomach pain he had talked to me about frequently over the previous nine years. He wasn't sure if he had checked himself into the psych ward or if he had simply not resisted institutionalization. He did tell me that he had a hearing coming up to determine when and how he would be released, which likely meant that he had been certified and was not there voluntarily.

Terry asked me if I would come and visit him. He said he was very heavily sedated and bored. He was also lonely.

About a month earlier Terry showed up at the field office in a terrible state. I was very happy to see him because I had not heard from him for a long time. I had correctly assumed he had caught a more serious charge and was in jail for a longer stretch again. Since Terry was kicked out of St. Mary's in 2015 for dealing drugs, he had been in and out of jail frequently for various offences related to dealing and theft. When he was not in jail he stayed in a string of shelters, with long stretches sleeping outside. Occasionally he secured a room in a supportive housing building, but these stays were always short-lived due to altercations with building residents and staff.

I knew that Terry avoided seeing me when he became less able to take care of his physical appearance in the context of frequent shelter hopping and homelessness. He contacted me most often when he had a relatively stable place to stay or immediately after visits with his grandma in Surrey, where he was able to do his laundry and shower. Across the years I knew him Terry clung tightly to a vision of himself as a dapper, street-wise entrepreneur who impressed people with his flair for style. His fashion choices had become less flashy over the years. He no longer wore embellished T-shirts, jeans, and hats, opting instead for the fairly standard uniform of monochrome black track suits with running shoes. However, he continued to put effort into his appearance. It was therefore shocking to see him walk into the office that day wearing clothes that were visibly filthy. His face and arms were covered with cuts and obvious skin infections, and his eyes looked swollen. He had gained a large amount of weight. Beyond his appearance, Terry seemed to be emotionally fragile in a way that I had never seen from him before. He acknowledged all of it right away, apologizing profusely about his appearance, for the smell, and for not being able to look me in the eye while we talked. I just kept saying over and over again how happy I was to see him and asking how I could help. Could I take him somewhere, even just to get some food? Did he want to see our nurse, who could help him with his wounds and talk privately about any other care or support that we could connect him to today? I felt utterly useless. What could I offer him, really? He told me that he just wanted to sit and talk. He had heard that I was looking for him to discuss next steps in the photography project and had decided to come that day because the project was not something he wanted to give up on even though he was in a really bad place. I realized that the only meaningful things I could offer him, perhaps, were our friendship and our collaboration on something that still mattered to both of us.

I took out my laptop and pulled up his photographs. I told him again what a great job he did on his photo essay. It centered on the places of his childhood, to which he still dreamed of finding his way back. Terry was reluctant to accept my praise, talking instead about how he could have worked harder on the project, could have done a better job. He broke down and started to cry. Eventually he told me that his relationship with his family had deteriorated to the point that he was no longer allowed to step foot on their property. The last time he went by his family home he saw a worker in the backyard, mixing cement for a new walkway. Terry was devastated because this was simple work that he knew how to do from his days working construction, and he would have been thrilled to be asked to do it by his dad and stepmom. But they did not ask him. Instead, when his dad had caught him looking into the backyard over the fence, he came outside and asked Terry to leave immediately. I recalled a journal entry about his family that Terry had shown me once in his room at St. Mary's. On a single page he had written the following lines in large, childlike letters: "Certain bridges have been broken and are not fixable. We may not realize this yet. But there is damage that can't be undone."

Terry's family asked him many times to go to detox and then residential treatment. They eventually told him that entering a residential treatment program was a condition for being in their lives and receiving their support. However, Terry never seemed to find his way there. Between methadone and his antipsychotic injection, Terry had been *on* treatment fairly consistently across the years I knew him. I often accompanied him when he went to take his methadone at a local pharmacy close to our field office. But Terry didn't take methadone with the goal of remaining abstinent from other opioids, as his family would have liked. He told me many times that he took it because, along with illicit opioids, it helped to relieve his crippling stomach pain and lessened the dopesickness when he found himself without money and drugs. He also told me that methadone and his antipsychotic injection were a big part of what kept him from "never being happy" and stuck in his current circumstances. Over the years Terry often commented that he felt more energized when he fell off his methadone for several days and was forced to restart his prescription at a lower dose (e.g., from 150 to 30 milliliters). A high dose of methadone combined with his antipsychotic injection left him feeling lethargic and unmotivated.

That day in the field office he reflected, "Between the methadone and the antipsychotic, I'm scared that I'm going to wake up one day and have no emotions. They are trying to fry my—labota—like kill my frontal lobe. When I come off my methadone though, and drop a hundred mils or whatever, I get this spunky feeling in me that I *want* to go to work and I want to get back on the job scene. I actually start showing up at the job place [a local temporary work agency] and picking up jobs." Terry admitted that during the previous year he had started shooting more meth to "properly wake himself up" and stay awake so that he could make the money he needed each day.

Terry wanted desperately to work. But before he could do that he was adamant that he needed surgery to address his stomach pain. Tears dripped off his nose and onto the floor as he described what it felt like. He knew that everyone—his family, numerous doctors, providers, and workers—thought that the pain was all in his head, that it was an aspect of his diagnosed schizophrenia. Terry went back and forth on whether he identified with this diagnosis. That day in the field office he was adamant that he was not mentally ill. The stomach pain was real. In fact, it was the most real thing in his life because it was the thing that determined all of the other things that he knew he needed to change and yet somehow could not. The stomach pain was the reason that he needed to use so much fentanyl and methadone and the reason that he needed meth to wake up. It was the reason he ended up in jail because he needed to make money for fentanyl, the thing that could take the pain away completely. And it was the reason he could not go to detox and residential treatment because without fentanyl the pain would simply be too much. The stomach pain was the reason that he lost his temper with increasing speed, got into altercations with building staff and residents when he was moved into supportive housing, and was kicked out onto the street. It was the reason he could not get what he wanted and needed most: a job as a longshoreman or a construction worker. Without the stomach pain he would be able to get off disability welfare and start saving money for a real apartment and a motorbike. He would be able to reconnect with his family and go around to their place for Sunday dinners again.

I offered many times to go with Terry to the specialist appointments that he assured me were happening related to his stomach pain, but he never took me up on the offer. I eventually concluded that whether or not his pain was real or medically solvable was none of my business. What was my business—what Terry was telling me again and again—was that all of his anxieties about the past, present, and future were bound to the feeling that there was something inside of him that hurt badly and wouldn't let him breathe. "I can't get a real breath in," he told me that day, attempting to demonstrate. The pain wouldn't let him move. "I can't even lift things anymore," he said. And the pain wouldn't let him move on with his life: get clean, physically recover, get a job, make things right with his family. He imagined that if the pain had never started his life would be dramatically different. He would have gotten out of the system, "made a man of himself." But because of it maybe he never would.

Two days after Terry messaged me from the psych ward I went to visit him there. I took the elevator up to the second floor of St. Paul's Hospital and buzzed the intercom to be let through the double-locked doors. As soon as I walked in I saw him standing there, waiting for me. His head had been completely shaved and he was wearing brown hospital scrubs. His face was round and noticeably free of cuts.

We had exchanged some Facebook messages earlier that day. Terry had told me how excited he was that I was coming to visit him. He had thanked me for my friendship over all these years, for the visits while he was in jail and now in the hospital, in a place that was not unlike jail. In Terry's case the similarities had nothing to do with institutionalization, with rules and locked doors, white walls and neon lights. Rather, for Terry, both jail and the psych ward offered a break, of sorts, from the everyday emergencies of his life on the streets. They provided a break shaped by the kind of total physical, psychological, and emotional exhaustion that made anywhere at all better than "out there." He desperately needed some kind of change, and this was what was available.

As we walked down the hall of the unit together toward a lounge where we could sit and talk, I could see that Terry was sedated and weary. In one of his hands he carried a small, disposable plastic Dixie cup of two-percent milk—the kind with the foil lid that needs to be carefully peeled back so that nothing spills out of the cup. In his other hand he clutched tightly the baseball cap and kale chips that I had brought for him at his request. When he showed me his room on the way down the hall I saw a half dozen or so other empty milk cups on his bedside table. Terry had told me at the field office a month earlier that he was hungry all of the time. Starving, and also perpetually empty, no matter how much he ate.

In the lounge we each took a seat on squeaky, acrylic chairs. There was a TV on one wall and a mural depicting a field of yellow flowers giving way to majestic, snow-capped mountains on another. Terry opened his kale chips and started eating, but he could barely stay awake once he was sitting down. He told me that they were heavily medicating him but that he had managed to cheek (not swallow) some of his meds and flush them down the toilet. He complained that he still did not have permission to go outside for smoke breaks, despite being good all weekend. He admitted that his temper had been getting the best of him and that the psychiatrist had started stationing a security guard by her office door during their meetings in case Terry became violent. He described the security guards as vicious, wild animals who wanted to tear into his flesh. What Terry really wanted to talk to me about, however, was his stomach pain. He had also become increasingly convinced that there were insects in his ears and growing out of his hair follicles. He was confused, frustrated, and angry that no one would take his health complaints seriously. "No one will listen to me," Terry mumbled. "I'm just another Native kid in pain to them."

I listened patiently to Terry, unsure, as I often was, of how to respond to what he was telling me. With all the young people I had grown close to over the years I wanted to be firmly on their side, to support them completely. Also, between Terry's last visit to the field office and what he was telling me that day in the psych ward, I believed that he was trying to articulate something vitally important about how systemic racism and entrenched marginalization and exclusion *felt*, in his mind and in his body. And yet I could also clearly see and hear signs of physical and mental illness.

As I got ready to leave I clumsily tried to convince him to use the time on the ward to rest, eat well, and take a break from intensive fentanyl and meth use. I implored him to be careful with fentanyl once he was allowed smoke breaks, as I knew how easy it was to procure and use drugs on or nearby the hospital grounds. And then, out of sheer desperation and the sense that I was leaving him with nothing but the most general, impersonal advice, I reached into my own memories from counselling sessions and online self-help blogs for something more meaningful to suggest. I told him about this idea I had heard of about "breaking up with your illness." Could he move forward with some aspects of his life, despite the pain and discomfort? To my surprise, he connected immediately to the idea. He started talking animatedly about how much he wanted a girlfriend, someone who understood what he was going through. We started talking about Laurie and her husband (although there was no official paperwork) Kevin, and how they seemed to be there for each other even though they were each dealing with very difficult things in their lives.

"They're made for each other," Terry said wistfully. "I would give absolutely anything to have something like that. I'd love to meet a girl like that. We could fall in love and have kids. We could get each other out of the life. I could help her, and she could help me."

Two years after this encounter in the psych ward, Terry died from an overdose. Perhaps because of the COVID-19 pandemic I learned of his death only many months later through an online obituary forwarded to me by a mutual acquaintance. I felt tremendous grief at the loss of this kind and gentle young man, who had taught me so many things over the years. I tried to imagine Terry free from the pain that had increasingly seemed to define his life. I tried to imagine him finding his way home, just as he had always wanted.

THE WAY HOME, TERRY, 2011

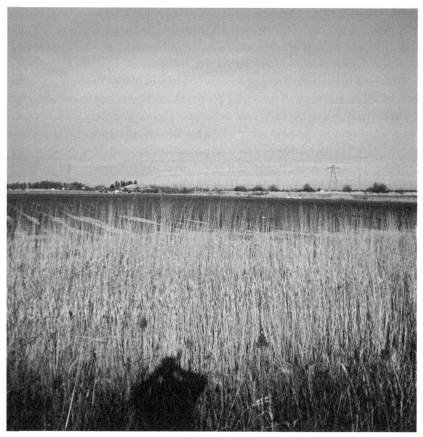

LAURIE, DOWNTOWN, 2018

In early 2018 Laurie began to tell me that the doctors in the hospital had stolen her baby. She left message after message about it on my phone and told me the story each time we ran into each other downtown or at the field office. She said that she planned to contact the media and sue the hospital. She asked me in vague terms to help her but never actually allowed me to make calls or visit a doctor with her so that I could better understand what had happened.

I saw Laurie several times in late 2017 with a visibly swollen belly. But she had never mentioned a pregnancy, and I never asked. Pregnancies came and went frequently among the young people I knew, and acknowledging them could be extremely sensitive. Pregnancies could engender a desired sense of forward momentum; they ignited the moral worlds in which young people were enmeshed and dreams for a different kind of life. But they also often prompted a state of suspension; they were feared and outright ignored. Pregnancies could end abruptly, including in the later stages, and swollen bellies could remain for a period of time in their absence. I therefore always waited to see whether and how young people would talk about pregnancies before asking any questions myself.

It never became clear to me whether Laurie was pregnant in 2017 or what happened in the hospital. Her husband Kevin remembered the incidents that Laurie was describing quite differently. He told me when we had a moment alone one time that he remembered being present for an ultrasound when the doctors explained to Laurie that she had a large cyst in her stomach, which would need to be removed surgically.

Laurie's story looped around and around. It was both well drawn out and fragile, like it might break apart if Kevin or I questioned her too aggressively. Neither of us wanted to do this. Kevin and I both knew that what was happening with Laurie could be interpreted as psychosis, as madness. Laurie did admit to me that she had recently been in the psych ward at St. Paul's Hospital after a Mental Health Act apprehension. I also knew that, since 2016, she had been living in supportive housing designated for individuals with concurrent disorders. But Laurie also continued to insist that she was not mentally ill or in psychosis as a result of many years of intensive meth use. She also refused the language of trauma, even as the services and systems she was navigating surely tried to interpret her life through this frame.

Anthropologists and activists, too, might want to interpret Laurie's story about her stolen baby as a manifestation of intergenerational trauma. Laurie did have a baby once, and that baby was taken away. She had been apprehended from her own mom by the state when she was a baby, and her mom (whom I also knew well by 2018) told me that she had been removed from her family as a child. Over the years I watched Laurie and her mom nurture their relationship into something more solid than it had been in the past. When she was younger and moving through various foster homes Laurie said that she had often felt abandoned by her parents and angry with them for failing to protect her against her abusers. But over the past several years, living in supportive housing buildings only a few blocks from each other in the Downtown Eastside, Laurie and her mom had grown closer and it was obvious how deeply they cherished the bond that they had been able to create after the violence of the past. Laurie's story about her stolen baby seemed to bring them even closer. On several occasions I witnessed Laurie's mom stoking its fire, encouraging Laurie to take on the doctors responsible for what had happened. It was a way for them to talk, perhaps, about things that had happened in the past and were still happening in the present that were fundamentally wrong and about something important that got abruptly ripped away.

As Laurie and her mom inhabited the story with growing ferocity, they did not seem miserable or heartbroken. Instead, they seemed energized and charged up as they told and retold the details of what had happened and could happen next. The story was about profound loss, but it also seemed to be full of optimism and desire. It was about what could possibly be gotten back and about building a family. It was about all four of them—Laurie, Kevin, their child, and Laurie's mom—being on the edge of a big change.

Kevin stayed firmly outside the story, often making it clear when we were all together that he would much rather flail off somewhere than listen to it again. Sometimes he did leave. But most of the time he stood or sat there silently, nodding occasionally, supporting the young woman he referred to as his wife. Twisting the ring on his finger that matched the one Laurie wore, he did not argue with or contradict her, even though he remembered things differently. Maybe, like me, he was uncertain of the truth of the matter and had determined that the truth was not what mattered here at all.

AARON, BEACHWOOD HOTEL, 2019

By late 2017 Aaron was spending most of his time at the Beachwood Hotel. He still officially had his own room in a nearby supportive housing building, but he rarely went there. Instead, he crashed in his friend Gerry's room at the Beachwood whenever he needed sleep. Aaron told me during our last recorded conversation in early 2019 that he wasn't sleeping or eating much anymore. "Just enough to stay alive," he said in a soft but steady voice.

Aaron was disappearing into his fentanyl use and spent endless hours playing Xbox in the room that he and Gerry essentially shared at the Beachwood. He had become even thinner, and his voice seemed quieter. I was struck by how little space he seemed to take up. It was almost as though he could sit there in the field office virtually unnoticed if it were not for my efforts to draw him out through conversation.

"My dope use is pretty out of control," he reflected, using the same language as he had in 2017 when he first became wired to fentanyl. There was no alarm in his voice. He said that fentanyl was better than meth at keeping away troublesome thoughts, and he had no intention of slowing down. He sounded so sure of himself. He said that he wasn't afraid of dying. Besides, he had yet to overdose.

As we talked I tried to imagine Aaron and Gerry sitting together in their small hotel room, faces lit by the glow of a large monitor and surrounded by piles of merch that Aaron said he continued to go out and move occasionally. Gerry was much older than Aaron. In 2019 Aaron was twenty-nine and Gerry was in his sixties. These kinds of friendships were not uncommon among the young men I followed. Aaron told me that Gerry looked out for him. He brought him food most days from the various drop-in services that Aaron so despised attending and went out and scored fentanyl for both of them when Aaron was stuck without money and drugs and lacking the energy to go out and hustle for both. There was care there and material support. Being tied to someone in this way eased the everyday emergencies of entrenched poverty and addiction (Bourgois and Schonberg 2009)—this could be as true for friendships as for romantic relationships. In fact, there could be a stability to friendships like the one between Aaron and Gerry that was absent from the romantic relationships I observed. I recalled that Aaron once told me he still wanted a big brother or dad in his life. His biological dad was "somewhere in the city," but they did not have a relationship as far as I knew.

From late 2017 to early 2019 Aaron seemed to find a sense of constancy with Gerry that he had not experienced previously, including throughout his years with Laurie. Whereas Laurie kept Aaron embroiled in the ups and downs of the various dramas between them, Gerry helped to ease Aaron into what seemed to be a welcome state of suspension. This was distinct from the crushing boredom described by so many of the young people I followed, in that a state of suspension—using fentanyl and playing Xbox endlessly, for example—did not necessarily demand release or action. Finally, Aaron was somewhere that he wanted to be, or at least he was no longer somewhere that he wanted desperately to get away from. For the moment he was not necessarily moving forward or backward, and there seemed to be relief in that for him. During this period I would occasionally see him and Gerry striding down Hastings Street in the Downtown Eastside, huddled close together and engaged in some private, conspiratorial exchange. They looked like family.

LULA AND JEFF, GREYSTONE HOTEL, 2019

In early 2019 I visited Lula and Jeff at the Greystone Hotel. They had been living there together for three years by that time, sharing Jeff's cramped single room (a large closet was how they often described it). Some of the things that Lula had up on the walls of her old room at Wenonah House had been transplanted to this new space, but the effect was less homey and more disjointed. As usual, Lula talked that day about how much she hated it at the Greystone, and Jeff talked about how what he really wanted was more space from Lula. It was his room, after all.

"The things is, I have nowhere else to go," Lula said flatly, as Jeff headed out the door to go score fentanyl and meth from his longtime dealer in the building.

Jeff was still using both fentanyl and meth, but not as intensively as he had been. He had recently gone on Kadian (slow-release oral morphine). After years of insisting he would never try OAT again, he said he had decided to try it after hearing from a friend that Kadian didn't have the same negative side effects as methadone or Suboxone—in fact, it produced a fairly pleasurable buzz and could really take the edge off dopesickness. Jeff was put on what he described as the highest possible dose, which was delivered to his door each morning at the Greystone. He told me that he had gradually reduced his use of fentanyl to three days a week and was reasonably happy with these changes. He didn't have to hustle as hard for money and drugs. He was getting fewer abscesses because he was injecting less. He had started working a few shifts in the overdose prevention site (OPS) in the Greystone, where he handed out harm reduction supplies, watched people use, and administered Narcan whenever there was an overdose. While he seemed happy to have the work, he said that everyone in the building now hated him because no one wanted to get Narcanned. Even as they accessed the Greystone's OPS, presumably to avoid a fatal overdose, they nevertheless wanted to experience that high that existed on the very edge of overdose, and on the very edge of death.

This was a line that Jeff himself walked for years, and Lula and I talked many times about how scared we were that Jeff would eventually overdose and die. Prior to 2019 he used more fentanyl than anyone else I knew. It therefore surprised me when Lula expressed ambivalence about Jeff's situation that day while he was out of the room scoring. She told me that these days Jeff often woke up, took his Kadian, and then slept for hours and hours on end. She said she was glad I was there because he was actually awake for a change.

"He's trying to slow down on the fentanyl, which is good, I guess," she sighed. "But when he's using more down [opioids], like, he'll get up and want to go get more and more. He has to go and make more money for it, panning or whatever. And he does that over and over and over. Sometimes he'll go out like five times a day. Come back here, you know, get more down, and then go out again. It's like, on repeat. But with Kadian he just takes it and sleeps all the time."

There was relief in Lula's tone, but also obvious frustration. She continued, "I feel like he's just wasting away now. You know what I mean? It's, like, great that he's not using as much. But he's not, like, *awake*. I don't want to say it, but I liked him better when he was using because at least he was up and active and talking to me. Instead of, like, sleeping. And I feel horrible saying that. Because of course I don't want him using down and overdosing. But at the same time, it's like, I end up getting bored. And then getting myself into trouble."

Across the years I witnessed repeatedly how Lula struggled to fill her time when she was not embroiled in the drama of her relationship with Jeff. Her meth use was intimately tied up with this drama. It fueled its intensity and helped to ameliorate the resulting emotional wounds. But meth was also something that helped Lula to navigate boredom when the drama receded for periods of time. When she and Jeff broke up, or when he was sleeping for long stretches, meth got her up and out and about on her old BMX bike, socializing with friends and new love interests across the downtown core. Lula tried to think through other ways to fill her time. She sometimes expressed the desire to get a part-time job, go to school, or work more wholeheartedly on her recovery. This usually happened when she and Jeff broke up and she was in a new romantic relationship with someone whose goal was to get clean and work. And while Lula continued to refuse to enter the treatment system again, occasionally she did detox herself off meth by taking her quetiapine and zopiclone and sleeping for several days at a time at a new boyfriend's place. But Lula told me that whenever this happened she soon felt the familiar weight of depression and boredom. The new boyfriends helped her to get clean, but they never seemed to be a route to the part-time job she desired. And so she went back to Jeff and to meth, repeatedly. The drama of that relationship once again expanded to encompass all of her time and energy, and she seemed to have nothing left to pursue other dreams. Except, that is, her role as a mom, which she clung to fiercely even as other parts of her life fell apart and came back together again and again.

Lula never did regain custody of her youngest daughter. She was adopted by the same foster family that had adopted Lula's other two children. But in 2019 Lula was allowed regular supervised visits most weeks. On these occasions her Facebook feed was flooded with images of the four of them together, smiling for selfies. The father of her youngest daughter also joined some of these visits, which pleased Lula. They were being parents to their daughter, even if it didn't look the way they once imagined.

In the spring of 2020 the COVID-19 pandemic hit Vancouver and Lula and Jeff became more isolated than ever in their closet-size room at the Greystone. Those few meal and drop-in programs that they did access were closed, and guests were no longer allowed inside supportive housing buildings. Lula's visits with her kids were cancelled. Boredom intensified, and for months the only lines of flight seemed to be intensive drug use or sleep. There was nowhere to go except deeper into drug use, somnolence, and the drama of their relationship, which was becoming increasingly violent.

During the pandemic I kept in touch with Lula and Jeff by phone. Even though Lula's relationship with her parents never fully recovered after her pregnancy and its aftermath in 2016 and 2017, they continued to pay for her phone. As a result she was one of the few young people I knew whom I could reliably get a hold of by phone and Facebook Messenger.

Throughout 2020 Jeff stayed on Kadian and Lula continued to hate how he behaved while on it. Jeff also eventually started taking hydromorphone tablets daily, which were prescribed to him as a risk mitigation measure during the overlapping COVID-19 and overdose public health emergencies (BC Centre on Substance Use 2020). Risk mitigation prescribing of pharmacotherapies such as hydromorphone and dextroamphetamine was intended to reduce risks and harms among people who use drugs by allowing them to better avoid withdrawal and overdose while socially distancing and self-isolating. Nevertheless, overdose rates soared to new heights during the first year of the pandemic (BC Coroners Service 2022), leading to increasing calls for a "real" safe supply of heroin, meth, and cocaine to curb the rising death toll (Drug Users' Liberation Front n.d.; Moakley 2021). Jeff acknowledged that he was still living on the edge of death, even as he remained on treatment. In early 2021 he was hospitalized following a life-threatening overdose.

"I'm still, like, rolling the dice, right?" he said to me over the phone a few weeks later. "Still playing Russian roulette, even though I'm on all these meds."

Jeff sounded resigned; Lula sounded increasingly angry. She had lost too many people by this point, and yet the deaths kept coming. From her perspective it was not just that she and her friends and loved ones were being left to die due to the absence of a safe supply of drugs. Lula seemed to increasingly distrust the professionalized housing, harm reduction, and research infrastructures that blanketed the active drug scenes in the Downtown Eastside and Downtown South neighborhoods. From her perspective the entire situation—from the drug scenes to the interventions that were purported to help people and save lives—was not rooted in compassion but in control and even annihilation. She refused to be drawn into the churn of intervention made even more frenetic by the declaration of the COVID-19 public health emergency, refused to live on the edge of change via risk mitigation prescriptions or even safe supply protests.

"They are slowly killing us off," she told me over the phone in 2021. "They decided to have another bad wave of dope going around." I tried to listen for who "they" might be. The government? But what Lula was critiquing seemed to go beyond that, to encompass every artery of downtown Vancouver's poverty management and public health infrastructures, from supportive housing building managers to harm reduction workers.

Lula continued, "I notice that every time one of my friends dies from fentanyl, no one can *ever* answer the question of where they got their dope from, and from who. Right? Nobody can answer that question. And I think they get those harm reduction workers or whatever to come and just hand them the dope. And they somehow get them to use it alone in—in their housing, or whatever. They *want* them to use alone so that they will die in their rooms alone. Like, especially on Welfare Day, when every building has a 'no guest policy'—it's just too easy."

Lula told me that she thought a lot about dying. "Most days, I feel like I can't do it anymore and I just—I just really want to go home, and be with Cody," she said. "But then I always hear his voice in my head saying, 'No, Lula, you need to stick it out. We will be together again one day, I promise you that. But, like, it's not now. You're still here for a reason.'"

Before Lula gave birth to her youngest daughter in 2017, one of her best friends, Cody, overdosed and died in his supportive housing room. Lula was devastated. She tried to come to terms with his death, even naming her daughter after him. Over the years that followed we talked about Cody frequently. Lula carried a printout from his celebration of life everywhere she went. Carefully smoothing the creased paper, she regularly showed me his photograph and obituary.

By 2021 so many young people were gone, and yet they were still around (Stevenson 2014). Lula couldn't let Cody go. And maybe, she told me, he couldn't let go of her either. She often sensed his presence and spent a lot of time talking to him. Eventually she started using an app on her phone to listen even more closely for messages from him from the spiritual world.

"One time, he said my name, so nice and clear: 'Lula,'" she told me again over the phone in 2021. I had heard this story countless times. The telling of it was perhaps a part of what kept Cody here, in this world, with her.

"And I'm like, 'Oh god, Cody, I miss you, I love you so much,'" Lula continued. "And he's like, 'I love you too and I miss you too.' And then this other voice came on, like, the voice of an Elder, a Native man. And he said, 'That's it.' And Cody was gone. And then the second time I heard him, he only said a few words: 'Lula, your daughter needs you.'" She paused. "And it's true, I'm still here, somehow. And I still have a purpose here, even if I don't totally know what that purpose is beyond, like, being here for my kids."

It seemed to me that the telling and retelling of this story was also, perhaps, a part of what kept Lula here too.

DOM, BC CHILDREN'S HOSPITAL, 2020

The churn of intervention to address mental health and addictions and overdose deaths in Vancouver continued unabated. In early summer 2018 the local children's hospital began piloting a new program for the increasing number of adolescents ages twelve to eighteen who were presenting in the emergency room following a life-threatening overdose. The program allowed these young people to be admitted to the hospital involuntarily—via, but also independently of, the Mental Health Act—for a period ranging from a few days to a couple of weeks. The goal was to prevent them from leaving the emergency room following the reversal of an overdose without any connection to treatment and care—from falling through the cracks of the healthcare system. During these "stabilization care" admissions, young people underwent a comprehensive medical and mental health evaluation and were connected with OAT (primarily oral and injectable buprenorphine-naloxone) if they consented to treatment.[2] They also often received treatment for concurrent medical and mental health issues, of which there could be many. Prior to discharge, follow-up treatment and after-care plans were developed via engagement with young people, biological family members, foster parents, social workers, and other stakeholders such as outreach workers and members of youth intensive case management teams.

The introduction of hospital-based stabilization care for young people who use drugs in Vancouver and elsewhere across BC generated fervent political activity among drug user and caregiver activists and policy makers on all sides of the issue. Many were deeply concerned about the steeply rising numbers of involuntary hospitalizations among young people in BC via the Mental Health Act (which increased by 162 percent between 2008 and 2018) and argued strongly that expanding involuntary approaches to care would ultimately do far more harm than good, particularly among young people who have experienced the violence of institutionalization across their lives and across generations (BC Representative for Children and Youth 2021; Goodyear et al. 2021; Pilarinos et al. 2018). Others argued that hospital-based physicians have a duty to protect these young lives, even if that means hospitalizing adolescents for periods of time against their will (Warshawski and Warf 2019). They suggested that the developmental characteristics of the teenage brain and frequent presence of concurrent mental health issues and cognitive disabilities, combined with the aftereffects of acute opioid intoxication, overdose, and administration of Naloxone, could significantly reduce adolescents' capacity to make independent, sound decisions regarding recommended treatment and care (Warshawski and Warf 2019). Following an overdose, many young people want to leave the hospital against medical advice. I witnessed this often. After receiving Naloxone, they are often in active withdrawal and experiencing intense cravings for opioids. Proponents of involuntary hospitalization argue that during this period an involuntary admission to hospital provides an essential "pause" that may restore young people's capacity to more fully understand the consequences of refusing recommended treatment and care. It also gives providers and caregivers time to figure out where they can go next, ideally to a longer-term treatment bed.

I understood the desperation that many providers at the local children's hospital felt—their desire to intervene, to do something, *anything*, to save these young lives, even in the short term. In many ways I shared it. In the context of a highly toxic drug supply, it was excruciating to stand there and watch young people walk away, knowing that they could be going to their deaths. Hospital-based providers were also under considerable pressure to intervene. By 2018 overdose was one of the leading causes of death among adolescents (BC Coroners Service 2018, 2022). But an older BC Representative for Children and Youth (2015) report, titled "Paige's Story: Abuse, Indifference and a Young Life Discarded," also seemed to fuel the will to intervene—at least in Vancouver. The Paige Report, as it was commonly known, had identified repeated hospital admissions as one of the "cracks" through which this young Indigenous woman had been allowed to consistently fall, until she died from a drug overdose in a public washroom in downtown Vancouver when she was nineteen. Across my fieldwork many of the providers I knew and interviewed—including those at the local children's hospital—were profoundly impacted by this report. They mentioned it recurrently as they contended with what their responsibilities were when it came to connecting young people with treatment and care.

I also understood the desperation of family members and caregivers who were arguing for involuntary hospital-based care. My own brother had overdosed and been hospitalized numerous times across my fieldwork. I knew intimately the relief that came when my family and I were informed that he would be held in the hospital involuntarily via the Mental Health Act because of concurrent mental health issues.

However, my research in and beyond institutional settings such as hospitals, supportive housing buildings, and residential treatment programs also showed me the lengths that some young people would go to in order to evade or escape from these places, often with devastating effects. I knew that even the threat of involuntary hospitalization could lead some to avoid calling 911 if someone was overdosing and needed help. It would drive some even further away from care— and not just hospitals—in an attempt to keep themselves safe from the often-times intimately familiar dangers of isolation, surveillance, and control. And then there was the still unanswered question of what was next for these young people, after their involuntary hospitalization, and after their connection to, and even completion of, a longer-term residential treatment program. Where did they go from there? Some could return to family homes, but many could or would not. For the latter, I saw that there continued to be a lack of stable, safe, and desirable housing, leaving many feeling that they were back at square one even when they were able to complete the plans laid out for them by various providers, workers, and teams.

In 2020, in the midst of this political maelstrom, I began a hospital-based ethnography of stabilization care admissions. I spent two days on the ward where adolescents were admitted before all research was shut down due to COVID-19. During those two days I met Dom, a charismatic, painfully tired sixteen-year-old, who perhaps initially tolerated my presence—in addition to a somewhat dizzying rotation of providers, workers, and visitors—and then eventually opened up to me because it was a way to pass the time until his admission was over.

Throughout 2020 and 2021 I attempted to continue my research on stabilization care admissions virtually. I spoke on the phone with all sorts of different kinds of providers involved in these admissions and with the biological and foster parents of the adolescents admitted. I was never able to speak to another young person admitted for stabilization care directly until I resumed in-person research in 2021. But during my phone calls with providers and caregivers I heard stories about them: about young people who were extremely agitated, yelling, swearing, and not making any sense, and about those who were utterly silent, who shut down completely. I could see familiar forms of evasion and refusal at play here, especially when I learned that the same young person who had been utterly incoherent or silent in front of providers then had a highly coherent visit with a trusted outreach worker or Elder.

Dom's reaction—or lack thereof—to his admission was different again, but equally familiar to me. He said that he probably wouldn't have stayed in the hospital if he had the choice, nor was he interested in refusing or resisting what was happening to him. "It's just something I have to get through," he said, yawning. Despite his fatigue, he paced around the room, unable to get comfortable on his hospital bed or in one of the encircling chairs. He continued, "I like this place a lot better than the other hospitals I've been in, so. They've got a big ass game room, a bunch of TVs, all these [video game] consoles. Just stuff to keep busy, which is nice, I guess."

Later in our conversation he elaborated, "I've, um, been in lots of situations like this. Juvie, jail, and stuff. I was in some kind of psych ward, I think? It was harder, before, when I was younger. I don't know. I was still adapting then, right? But now I know, uh, I really can't do anything about it."

Across his young life Dom had adapted to institutionalization. Now he seemed quietly resigned to passing this latest stretch without incident. Or maybe he was just so very, very tired. Dom told me he had been to so many different treatment programs already, to so many different drop-ins. None had worked. But this time, at this hospital, he was being offered one thing that was different: Suboxone. And while he wasn't sure if he could feel anything from it yet, he seemed modestly hopeful that it might be the thing that would allow him to get back to work, to get back to school, and to forge different kinds of relationships: "real" friends, a nice girlfriend. With a tone of cautious optimism and a small smile, he told me, "This time, I'm trying something a different way, I guess?"

Dom died from an overdose several months later in 2020.

CARLY AND CONNOR, FIELD OFFICE, 2018

Connor came into the field office in the spring of 2018 to tell me that Carly had died from an overdose. He was very matter of fact about her death, talking about it like he had been expecting it for a long time. I, on the other hand, was shocked by this news. By 2018 there were so many young people who I worried would die from an overdose. Each time I saw them I thought that it might very well be the last time. But I had never thought this about Carly.

In hindsight, that seemed stupid. By the time Connor had shown up at the field office that day in 2018, I had been unsuccessfully trying to get in touch with Carly for six months or so. This was highly unusual. Since we had met in 2008, I was always able to contact her by phone or Facebook Messenger. And then, quite suddenly in the late fall of 2017, I stopped hearing from her.

The last time I saw Carly was summer 2017. I spent the afternoon with her at her new market rental one-bedroom apartment in a residential neighborhood in the south of Vancouver. We sat on the floor of her living room for several hours, playing with her one-year-old son and small dog. The third-floor apartment was decorated in much the same way as her last place, except for the addition of various baby stuff and a small desk with a computer on it in one corner of the living room. The afternoon sun beat down on the west-facing windows. It was stiflingly hot inside, even with the sliding glass doors of a small balcony pushed open. Despite the heat and glowering stares we were receiving from her son's dad each time he went in and out of the apartment, Carly seemed happy and energized. She told me that she was no longer romantically involved with her son's dad but that he still came around a lot to spend time with their son. He continued to be abusive toward her, but she was handling it. She said that this time she was determined to "hold her life together" no matter what was going on with the men in her life. She owed it to her son to "just keep going" the way she had been since getting pregnant with him.

When Carly learned about her most recent pregnancy in 2015, she decided that this time she would do everything that the social workers were asking of her from the outset. During the pregnancy she attended a treatment program even though she was already two months clean when she began the program. She steadily distanced herself from Connor, who by 2016 was living in a supportive housing building downtown. Following the birth of her son in 2016, Carly remained at the local women's hospital for the requisite period of time and then moved into Fern Grove with her son to complete their residential program. From there the two of them moved in with her parents before finally getting the apartment where they were living in 2017 with the help of a BC Housing rent subsidy. Carly had also almost completed the weekly three-hour parenting course mandated by the Ministry of Children and Family Development. She informed me with pride that the social worker would soon be closing her son's file. In a matter of months the supervision order that had been in place since his birth would be lifted and she would have full custody. Recently she had even started to hope again that she might regain custody of her other two children as well, although she had not seen them in over two years. She was just about to celebrate two years clean.

As the afternoon turned to early evening and we said goodbye, I remember thinking to myself that Carly was inhabiting a version of the life she and so many others had longed for: she was living with her son in a "normal" apartment in a "normal" Vancouver neighborhood. They had a dog and played at a nearby park each day. Her son would start day care soon, and she planned to go back to school to become a drug and alcohol counselor. She said she wanted to help people who were where she had been for so many years.

Carly and I both so desperately wanted this to be the end of her story in terms of her involvement in my research. That last day we saw each other we discussed the photography exhibit, which I was beginning to plan. She told me that I could display her images, including one of a child's stroller sitting in the darkening backyard of her parents' house, taken so many years ago when she and Connor were actively trying to get their two children back from the ministry. Their photo essay was titled "Everything We Need." It meticulously documented the home-making project and elaborate geography of agencies and meetings that they were navigating in an effort to prove to the ministry that they could be good parents. Carly continued to be proud of this work, but I got the sense that the images reflected a mix of longing, anticipation, and anxiety that no longer characterized her sense of place in the city. She told me that day in her apartment that she hoped the images and the exhibit could help someone who was going through what she had gone through in the past. She said she may or may not be able to attend the exhibit depending on what was happening with her child care and schooling. I wondered whether our visits would continue, not because I was worried about her well-being but because she noted a few times during our conversation that she didn't think she had much more to offer me in terms of her participation in my research.

For a while after that visit to her apartment we kept in touch by phone and Facebook Messenger. She told me a bit about her school program. It seemed to be going well. And then she abruptly stopped messaging me or returning my phone calls. Eventually there was no more activity on her Facebook page. These kinds of "shadows and disappearances" (Meyers 2013, 5) were common; I often lost touch with young people for periods of time depending on what was going on in their lives. They went on and off Facebook, abandoned old profiles, and started new ones. Sometimes we lost touch permanently. I never pressed the issue. I thought it should be up to them if they wanted to remain in contact with me and involved in the research. But standing with Connor in the field office in

2018, having just learned about Carly's death, I wondered, should I have done more to keep in touch? Would it have made any difference to what happened?

Connor said that he never stopped worrying about Carly, even after they broke up and he watched her pull her life together for her son. He reflected angrily on how the main focus of the various professionals in their lives had always been *his* crack use and *his* mental health issues. Meanwhile, he watched Carly descend again and again into intensive opioid use, quietly destroying the marriage and family that he thought they were trying to build together. Carly's relapses often followed a predictable pattern. First, she started taking more methadone, either getting her dosage upped by her doctor or buying it on the street. Then she started using morphine on top of the methadone, and then heroin/fentanyl. She spent more and more time lying on the couch, sleeping. It was her favorite thing in the world, she told me many times over the years: that feeling of sedation, of melting into the couch.

Carly always hoped that her children, family, housing stability, and a daily routine could lift her out of the desire for long stretches of opioid-induced sleep that she said she had felt for as long as she could remember. She seemed to have those things in the summer and early fall of 2017. Perhaps, in the end, they weren't enough. Perhaps she just couldn't keep going. Maybe the abuse from her son's dad got really bad. Maybe school fell through. I'll never know. I suppose I cannot even know for certain that Carly is dead, only that she is gone. Gone from Facebook, gone from the phone number I had for her. Gone according to what Connor said in the field office that day, which was the last time I saw him. Connor was unable or unwilling to share more of the details of Carly's death or to contact her parents (whom I had met a few times over the years) so that we both might get some answers.

Connor told me he was ready to close that chapter of his life. He needed to finally get out of Vancouver. He liked the supportive housing building where he was living, but he wanted to get away from the ACT team and out from under the Extended Leave agreement he was on. He longed to get out of poverty and fantasized about large and small ways he might strike it rich—selling crack again or coming up with a brilliant invention that could be sold for millions. He also missed his mom terribly. As he was leaving the field office he insisted that this was the year to finally make that trip back home to Toronto that he had been dreaming about ever since Carly brought him out to Vancouver in 2007.

JOE, FIELD OFFICE, 2018

The last time I saw Joe was in our field office in winter 2018. I had seen him around since he and Patty broke up in 2015, and he occasionally called me from the office phone at the Greystone Hotel, usually at odd hours when it was impossible for me to pick up. His visit to me at the field office that day was a rare occurrence by then. He came in out of the rain, his track suit plastered to his alarmingly thin frame. He was smiling to himself, a wide-open, private smile about something only he knew about.

"Joe isn't really *here* anymore," Jeff had said during a recent visit with him and Lula. "But he seems happy," he added thoughtfully.

"Joe is a lost soul," Patty told me a few months earlier. The two of them continued to see each other occasionally, as she sank deeper and deeper into fentanyl use and he alternated between olanzapine-fueled somnolence and meth-fueled reveries. That day in 2018 Joe seemed to be in the latter state. He was jumpy and giggly, his legs bouncing rapidly against the chair he was sitting on. He agreed to do a more formal, audio-recorded interview with me in one of the private rooms. I think I knew that this could be one of our last chances to have this kind of conversation.

During this last interview Joe reflected on the string of mental health crises that he had experienced immediately before and after breaking up with Patty. Often, he had been picked up by police at the Lakeshore Hotel and then at the Greystone and taken to St. Paul's Hospital for assessment. Then he would be returned to his building, where he was sure he could hear the voice of his biological mom echoing through the hallways. "It was kind of nice," he said. "To hear her there. I miss her so much. It's not all bad, when that happens." He remembered nothing of his breakup with Patty, including who had broken up with whom. "I was barred from the Lakeshore, and I think we just saw each other less and less," he shrugged. "And now I just miss her lots. I just miss my friend. That's about all I have to say about that."

Joe said that eventually he was "coerced" into taking olanzapine, which began being delivered to his door at the Greystone each day by a member of an adult mental health team. He was put on Extended Leave; failure to take his meds would result in rehospitalization. After taking his olanzapine, Joe said that he would often sleep the entire rest of the day away, these long periods of slumber occasionally punctuated by long periods of wakefulness achieved through the intensive use of meth. He liked getting a lot of sleep. But meth seemed to be the only thing that could wake him up.

Joe seemed to want to be elsewhere—elsewhere in the city, elsewhere within the landscape of his own mind. The drugs took him elsewhere, took him everywhere. On meth he traversed the city, scavenging for cans. He heard the voices of loved ones who were far away or gone. He said he wanted to be moved back into the Lakeshore, even though the Greystone was "the exact same kind of supportive housing place." He wondered if going to detox for a week could be an effective bargaining chip in terms of making that move happen. Joe told me that, even without Patty's nagging, he still went to detox about once or twice a year in order to balance out and gain some weight. He believed that gaining weight in particular increased his tolerance for fentanyl and meant that he wouldn't overdose as easily. Joe still used opioids whenever he had extra money, in particular on Welfare Day. He told me he had overdosed twenty times in the last year, at least. I knew from Patty that one of these overdoses happened in her room. She and Joe had gone to the Salvation Army for Christmas dinner together. Patty brought him a bunch of neatly wrapped gifts. After dinner they went back to her room at the Lakeshore (by that time Joe had been un-barred) to use some fentanyl, and Joe had gone down. He had to be Narcanned four or five times.

Before he left I reminded him gently, "I'm always here to help. If you need help, you can call me." He left the field office still smiling to himself. But he never returned one of my phone calls ever again, even when I called him back in 2018 when I learned that Patty had died.

PATTY, EVERYWHERE, 2018

The last time I saw Patty was during the opening night of the photography exhibit. The vacant storefront we rented in downtown Vancouver was packed with people. About half of those who had been involved in the project managed to show up and invited various friends, family members, cherished outreach workers, and other frontline service providers. Many of my colleagues were also there, and my own family and friends. Trix wore towering patent stilettos, a full-length sequined green gown, and big hair. Lula and Jeff showed up at the beginning of the night in the midst of a huge argument. Lula was sobbing, and she and I had to go outside together until she was calm enough to come back in. But when I looked around the room later in the evening I saw her and Jeff standing close together under their professionally framed photographs, talking happily to Lula's parents. Laurie and Kevin were also there, as animated about the project as I had ever seen them. To the surprise of everyone there who knew her, Laurie even made a short speech during the point in the evening when we invited everyone to talk briefly about their photographs. I was equally surprised when Aaron showed up toward the end of the evening, giving me a silent nod of approval when he saw his framed photographs. He stayed well away from Laurie and Kevin.

Others were there and not there. Photographs of the city taken by Jordan, Lee, Carly, Terry, Janet, Patty, and Joe across the previous seven years hung on the walls, full of beauty and filth, longing and despair. During the welcome provided by a Nisga'a Elder, we remembered Jordan and Lee and Carly, and so many others who had lived and died young in Vancouver.

Patty and Joe's photograph of a local beach during wintertime, empty except for a single anonymous figure standing close to the icy water, was everywhere.

We had chosen it for our promotional materials. It was printed on the front of every postcard and brochure that littered the tables around the room, and it hung on the wall. And then, suddenly, Patty herself was there, standing in the doorway. I was on the other side of the room and immediately started pushing my way through the crowd to get to her. She took a few steps inside. I saw that Jeff was smiling at her, waving her over to come and join him and Lula. But I could see from Patty's face that she was overwhelmed, that it was all too much. Before I could make it halfway across the room she turned and left. I went out into the street to try and catch her, but she was gone.

A couple of months before the photography exhibit Patty and I met up in her neighborhood for coffee. She was thinner than I had ever seen her, wearing gray leggings and an oversize hoody. She had dyed her hair bright orange and was wearing it in a high, stringy ponytail. Her mood was erratic that day, and she jumped quickly between seemingly disparate thoughts. One minute she was upbeat and chatty, and the next she was in tears and unable to find any words at all.

There was the usual endless drama to recount. Patty told me in animated detail about how the guys she brought back to her room were always trying to crash with her, taking her stuff and sharing her drugs without reciprocating, and seemed to eventually "all have the same ideas" about her going out and making money for them through sex work. One guy left a whole bunch of particularly lucrative merch in her room, which slowly but surely disappeared as Patty and her friends sold it off, resulting in a debt that Patty then had to work to pay off.

On the one hand, Patty talked about how she "liked the challenge" of these sorts of situations. She was looking for a new boyfriend and wanted to find someone who was daring and exciting. On the other hand, I got the sense that the drama of her life had turned darker, more violent, and even deadly. In the last few months one of her potential boyfriends came over with a loaded gun. She was getting hit a lot. A guy had overdosed and died in her room, another in her hallway. The latter had also started out in Patty's room. She told him firmly that she didn't have any Narcan, that she would not Narcan him if he went down. She managed to push him out of the door before he fell to the floor. The building staff and paramedics tried to help him, but he didn't make it. Patty told me that she was so incredibly sick of people going down, and of Narcanning them, even as she recognized that her own two recent overdoses had been reversed by Naloxone. People were dying all around her, she told me, whether by overdose, suicide, or violence.

Patty seemed to be trying to ignore much of what was going on around her. But she also told me that she felt ignored, as though everyone had "given up on her." I asked her whom she meant.

"Just people," she replied. "Friends. My family. Service places." She started to cry. "I still think I'm a good person, you know? But it seems like less and less people are seeing that in me."

During the darker moments of our conversation that day Patty seemed to be working through whether she was going to give up on herself in certain ways. She told me that she wanted to get a CAT scan of her brain, to see how much damage her many years of intensive meth use had caused. When she was thirteen, at the first drug treatment program she had ever attended, she was shown a documentary about a boy who used meth. "They did a CAT scan and he had holes in his brain. From the crystal. Smoking it puts holes in your brain, and, like, injecting it kills your organs. And lately, I'm wanting to get my own scan because I'm wondering, like, am I *ruined*? Have I ruined my brain for good—like, permanently?"

I asked her about going to treatment and whether she ever thought about that anymore. Patty had been off OAT for years at this point. She said methadone reminded her of Joe, of the countless times the two of them went to the pharmacy together to drink their juice. She also hated the way methadone made her feel, and not feel. She wanted to experience the immense, otherworldly rush of fentanyl, not the more subdued buzz of methadone.

"I don't really think about treatment anymore," she replied. "Because, like, the thing is, I, like, never see treatment working out for people. For the people down here who are like me." Then she continued more thoughtfully, "The thing is that Joe and I would take breaks together. Sometimes we would just sleep and sleep, right? But now it's like, I don't have anyone to take breaks with. So, it seems like since they've taken Joe away from me, I've really been going downhill. Like, I don't sleep anymore. I've gotten myself so, so hooked on this down—this fentanyl. It's so much more addictive than heroin, I guess? I'm just like completely, totally focused on my down addiction at this point. And then with the meth, I don't do as much as I used to but, like, people like me, who have ADHD really badly? Like the meth is almost like a prescription medication. I used to be on Ritalin, right, but my doctor here would never give it to me. So, I need that shot [of meth] each day."

Patty had been doing sex work again since she and Joe had broken up, but it was no longer bringing in enough money to support her fentanyl use. She had started boosting and told me it was only a matter of time before she was arrested. "I just, like, don't know how to make everything in my life work right now. How do I make it all work?" she asked me tearfully.

Patty seemed to have sunken down into something so large and powerful that, in certain moments at least, there no longer seemed to be any clear directions out. The size and intensity of her addiction seemed to confuse as much as overwhelm her. In the past Patty referred to her and Joe as lost within the maze of institutions that they were trying to navigate, but I never saw the two of them that way. From my perspective they were anchored to each other, and I believed that would be enough for them to make some kind of life together in the city. But that day in the café Patty did seem lost to me, because she seemed lost to herself.

As she struggled through the most difficult moments of our conversation, I noticed that she still reached for Joe, for the memories of their time together that might provide some kind of anchor, or at least a sense of peace. Patty recalled, "Amazingly enough, the spot where I'm working [doing sex work], Joe was the first one to show me it. Joe was the one who got me into prostitution here, because he was doing it. He was working in Boys' Town when we first met up here. And then I got him out of that life, and he got me out of it, and we saved each other like that, over and over and over again." She paused for a long time. "The last time I saw him, I tried to tell him, like, it's okay that we broke up, because you and me spent enough time together for a lifetime. We made a lifetime of memories. We had a whole life together."

Before we said goodbye I asked Patty if she still wanted me to keep calling her. It had been so hard to contact her during the previous few years, and I worried that she no longer enjoyed, or at least got some benefit from, our time together. I remembered the days when we had spent hours and hours together, talking and dreaming about the future. Things seemed so different now. Patty told me she did want me to keep calling her. I told her she could call me anytime if she needed help, or just wanted to talk. She assured me that she would, but we never spoke again.

Not long after the photography exhibit my own life moved on in significant ways. I got pregnant and had to take large periods of time away from work due to a difficult pregnancy. Then I went on parental leave. Then the COVID-19 pandemic began. I tried to stay in touch with as many young people as I could by phone and Facebook Messenger, but Patty never returned any of my calls.

I did stay in touch with Lula and Jeff, and it was the two of them who sent me a Facebook message in 2020 to tell me that Patty had died. I called them immediately and learned that rumors were already swirling about the true cause of Patty's death.

Patty had overdosed, but she had not just overdosed.

Patty had an allergic reaction to something in her dope.

Maybe Patty had not overdosed at all.

Patty had increasingly seemed like she *wanted* to overdose, like she wanted leave this place, like she was ready to go.

Because of the COVID-19 lockdown there was no memorial for Patty at the Lakeshore Hotel. Instead, for about two months following her death Lula, Jeff, and I called each other to talk about Patty and to remember her, just as we had once done with Lee. Every so often I took flowers down to the beach that she had photographed all those years ago, which she told me symbolized everything that she loved about the city, everything that she was dreaming of in Vancouver. A place for her and Joe within its stunning beauty and promise.

WHERE WE'VE ENDED UP, PATTY AND JOE, 2013

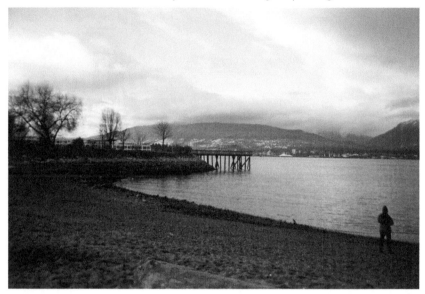

AFTERWORD

This is a book about endings: the endings of young people's lives, of their relationships to one another, and to place. But it is also about lives and stories that continue to be in motion, perhaps even when it comes to those who are gone. Rayna, Lee, Jordan, Laura, Tom, Terry, Dom, Cody, Carly, and Patty are remembered and missed. Their stories and words live on in this book, where perhaps they may have some impact. Sometimes it seems like a part of them is still here, in this world, communicating with those they loved and who loved them. At the time of writing, to the best of my knowledge, all of the other young people who populate these pages are still alive. The dreams of place they shared with me so many years ago have been irreparably altered by their trajectories in the city. But they live on, dreaming new dreams.

Those I came to know do not perhaps fit easily within the prescriptions of many policy makers and providers, nor the academic ideals of some critical scholars. They did not want to be framed as the damaged victims of overlapping forms of structural oppression, nor as intrepid underdogs resisting historical and ongoing injustices. Let me state clearly here that many important stories of resistance and activism can be told about people who use drugs in Vancouver, as individuals and communities, and in particular Indigenous individuals and communities, continue to demand change on terms that exceed pathologizing and criminalizing framings (Boyd, MacPherson, and Osborn 2009; Culhane 2003; Lupick 2017; Martin and Walia 2019). These stories of activism and resistance include young people who use drugs (Canêdo et al. 2022). This, however, is a different kind of story. It is a story about a group of young people who longed to belong and become in a city they loved, and who made fragile homes and families with each other there for a time. It is a story about how even the most progressive, made-in-Vancouver drug and housing policies sometimes fail because they do not adequately account for these lives, dreams, and desires, nor do they open up meaningful possibilities for these to flourish (Dorries 2019). Instead, policies and programs continue to be dictated by the categories and ideals of policy makers, providers, workers, police officers, researchers, and other professionals, even as calls for youth-focused and youth-friendly services and programs abound.[1]

Those I followed generally refused to be named and confined according to these categories and ideals, whether via the public health language of mental health and addictions or the more activist-oriented language of harm reduction. They rejected the lines we might want to draw between us and them, insisting on their inclusion in broader civic ambitions and imaginaries of the cosmopolitan city. Or they simply wanted to keep us guessing (and perhaps themselves as well) about who they were and where they were going next. Across this project new spatializations of power continuously worked to create docile bodies (Foucault 1997b). Settler colonialism was a "living phenomenon" (Monture 2007) that contained, displaced, and disappeared Indigenous bodies through new imbrications of care and control (Coulthard 2014; Razack 2015; Stewart and La Berge 2019). Simultaneously, new forms of life and refusal always emerged and exceeded these efforts.

Young people refused to reduce Vancouver's livability and promise to living in supportive housing, getting and staying on treatment, or accessing harm reduction programs. They wanted more than that. As time passed, however, it felt to many like that was all they were being offered. In this context it seemed to me that the question of how best to live on was answered first and foremost affectively: if they could not be bound to life by the momentum and future possibilities of school, work, parenting, and homemaking, they nonetheless could be bound to life by the more immediate momentum and sensorial possibilities of intensive substance use. Day after day, the drama of drug use, dealing, debts, crime, and romantic relationships propelled them forward, even as they generated significant suffering and harm.

Policy makers and providers are very interested in better understanding the *effects* of different programs and services but may neglect the extent to which these are registered and evaluated *affectively*. They could get young people moving forward with their lives or hold them back, make them feel like they were stuck again or that they were somehow getting lost. As Lauren Berlant (2011) so persuasively argues, affect served as a leading, visceral indicator of both threat and promise, oftentimes simultaneously. Senses of momentum and stagnation and a churn of stops and starts moved through and accumulated in places, dreams, bodies, relationships, substances, and pharmacotherapies. Attending to these rhythms and intensities and how they traveled and transmuted to produce particular affective geographies was crucial to understanding the forms of life, death, and harm emerging among this group of young people in Vancouver.

Of course all our lives are characterized by "rhythms of flow and arrest" (Stewart 2007, 19) that alternatingly drive us forward and hold us in place. In many ways this is what it means to be human in the "crisis ordinary" of the contemporary moment (Berlant 2011, 8). The difference, perhaps, lies in whether these rhythms ultimately take us somewhere—anywhere—that we want to go. This book reframes marginalization and vulnerability affectively; for those I followed, these seemed to be inextricably bound up with an inability to get somewhere better despite constant, grinding efforts to move forward and the seemingly endless churn of intervention occurring all around them. There was, for many, no desirable exit. I contribute to previous discussions about the ongoing effects and affects of settler colonialism (Million 2013; Stevenson 2014) and the settler-colonial city (Dorries et al. 2019; Peters and Anderson 2013), casting a disturbing light on Indigenous young people's felt knowledge of colonialism and how it shaped the recurring forms of loss operating on the bodies of the Indigenous future (Garcia 2010). I also shed light on how and under what terms Indigenous young people make urban space and place (Dorries 2023; Dorries et al. 2019; Peters and Anderson 2013), bringing into view more ambivalent—but no less powerful—forms of Indigenous life, flight, and refusal in the city that are not necessarily encompassed by narratives of resistance or contestation or even community. I hope I have raised fundamental questions about the cities we live in and what we are collectively becoming, as those in the margins are trapped, dislocated, and disappeared through new imbrications of crisis and care, and subjected to new or deepening forms of physical, psychological, emotional, social, economic, and spiritual injury. The answer is challenging, and very troubling.

NOTES

INTRODUCTION

1. I use the terms "addiction" and "addicted" carefully, recognizing that many people object to their etymology—the earliest usage of this language in Roman law referred to a state of slavery—and modern connotations (Gomart 2002). However, those I followed regularly used this language to describe the magnitude of what they were contending with, and I do not want to sanitize the intensity of their substance use or the frenetic cycles of use, withdrawal, and procurement that characterized their daily lives. This language was also regularly employed institutionally by policy makers and providers.

2. Vancouver is consistently ranked among the world's most livable cities across categories such as stability, health care, education, infrastructure, culture, and environment (Economist Intelligence Unit 2022).

3. Gilles Deleuze and Felix Guattari's thinking on the openness and flux of social fields can be helpful for making sense of worlds that are always in motion, drawing our attention to the dynamic trajectories of young people's lives (Biehl and Locke 2017a; Deleuze 2006). The notion of a line of flight takes two forms in Deleuze and Guattari's thought: *ligne de fuite* and *lignes d'erre*. While the former evokes "the act of fleeing or eluding but also flowing, leaking, and disappearing" (Deleuze and Guattari 1987, xvii), the latter refers to wanderings and reimaginings of geography. While both of these conceptualizations can be meaningfully brought into conversation with my ethnography, I find the former articulation (*ligne de fuite*) particularly helpful for understanding moments when individuals exceeded or broke through apparently rigid social formations and fields, opening up new possibilities (see also Biehl and Locke 2017a).

4. Single room occupancy hotels (SROs) are multiple-tenant buildings that house one or two people in individual rooms. They were originally built to meet the lodging and entertainment needs of Vancouver's seasonal and almost exclusively male workers. Rooms are typically three meters by three meters in size, with shared bathroom and kitchen facilities. During my fieldwork, SRO rooms were rented either by a landlord or the state as permanent, low-income residences for around $375 per month. Rent was commonly deducted directly from monthly social assistance (welfare) payments, leaving those who received regular social assistance with around $235 to live on per month. All dollar figures throughout are Canadian dollars.

5. Anishinaabe scholar Heather Dorries (2023, 117) defines Indigenous urbanism as "the dialectical relationship between Indigeneity and urbanism, marking both as formations that are constantly in flux and open to contestation.... [Indigenous urbanism] marks urban space as potentially liberatory and oppressive, oftentimes simultaneously."

6. In *Renegade Dreams: Living through Injury in Gangland Chicago*, Laurence Ralph (2014) similarly centers his interlocutors' dreams of place. We are both interested in how dreams and dreaming constitute a "conscious attempt to navigate one's place in the world" (2014, 193). In the Eastwood neighborhood that is the setting of his ethnography, Ralph (2014, 8) notes that these dreams often took the form of more "banal" desires for different kinds of futures (for example, the ability to walk to school safely), leading him to initially misrecognize residents' daily struggles as dreams. Among Eastwoodians, various physical, psychological, emotional, and economic injuries endowed these commonplace dreams with a renegade or defiant quality; "the power of such dreams [was] in having them and working toward them, regardless of

whether or not they [came] to fruition" (2014, 8). The dreams of place that I describe are different from those documented by Ralph in at least two ways. First, many of those I followed explicitly and rather provocatively articulated grandiose visions of the future—futures that involved buying and owning a house in Vancouver's exorbitant real estate market, for example, or going to the top-ranked University of British Columbia, or owning their own successful business. These were not renegade dreams born out of injury but rather demands for inclusion in widely shared urban imaginaries and challenges to prevailing assumptions about who these young people were and where they belonged. Second, I came to understand that young people's dreams, and the process of articulating them over and over again, were often less about working toward them in concrete terms than about propelling themselves forward day after day. Dreams and dreaming could engender particular affective intensities that included being at the center of something rife with potential, regardless of what actually transpired.

PART 1   DREAMS OF PLACE

1. As is standard practice in this research setting (Boilevin et al. 2018; Neufeld et al. 2019), young people were compensated financially for their participation in many aspects of this project (for example, participation in more formal, audio-recorded, in-depth interviews).

2. It has been suggested that the anxieties bound up in neoliberal capitalism—vast inequities and the gap between the real and the ideal, for example—find their most forceful expression in the predicament of youth (Comaroff and Comaroff 2000). Of course, too-easy analyses of capitalism and neoliberalism can obscure shifting and multiple realities on the ground (Tsing 2005); these are moving forces immanent in scenes, subjects, and places (Stewart 2007). However, the world over, young people who find themselves on the losing end of these processes seem to exist in local worlds that engender an uneasy mix of inclusion and exclusion. In this context, the city frequently emerges as a site for new claims.

3. In Canada, a reserve is a tract of land set aside under the Indian Act and treaty agreements for the use of Indigenous Peoples. Such land continues to be held in trust by the Crown and is subject to various permissions and inhibitions (Harris 2002). Reserves therefore continue to function as colonial spaces and powerfully shape the opportunities and movements of Indigenous people, including to places like Vancouver.

4. I use the term "clean" throughout this book with caution, recognizing its potentially stigmatizing connotations (i.e., the notion that substance use is "dirty"). However, this was overwhelmingly the language used by young people to differentiate between periods of abstinence from substance use and periods of intensive use.

5. While the field office is not technically a street youth service, young people rarely made this distinction.

6. The notion that the frictions of anthropological research can result in these moments of departure—for the researcher and also, perhaps, for the researched—resonates with the argument that it is often the research process itself that is the primary locus of value in contemporary anthropology, rather than our specific research questions and outputs (see also Castañeda 2005; Culhane 2011; Elliott 2014).

7. Stephen Collier and Andrew Lakoff (2005) define regimes of living as tentative and situated configurations of practices and practical knowledges, relationships and habits of relating, and technologies of administration and political elements that are brought into alignment in situations where the question of how to live is at stake. Young people simultaneously enacted multiple regimes of living that were continually reworked and reshaped across time in response to the shifting exigencies of particular situations. The regimes of living they enacted were often bound up with desires for things to be otherwise, or with a pained sense that they never would be for people like them.

8. Located in the adjacent province of Alberta, Fort McMurray is the heart of one of the oil production hubs in Canada.

9. Eugene Raikhel and William Garriott's (2013b) concept of addiction trajectories alerts us to how addiction as a lived experience, object of intervention, and category of thought throws people into new forms of life and harm that span intimate and institutional domains. Here, I am concerned with tracing how this directed movement—across places like shelters, SROs, supportive housing buildings, treatment and recovery facilities, and various elsewheres—opens up social, economic, spatial, and affective possibilities at the same time as it closes down others. Rather than reducing addiction and care to the workings of political economy, biopower, or governmentality, a focus on trajectories invites us to attend to both the "forces that structure and determine social phenomena into well-worn paths and those that maintain the contingency and indeterminacy of those paths, allowing individuals to veer off into unexpected directions" (Raikhel and Garriott 2013b, 8).

10. Embodied senses of place can be productively analyzed through Pierre Bourdieu's (1977, 1997) notion of habitus. Habitus is the incorporation of the social into the body; it reflects hidden forms of power but is frequently misrecognized as individual choice, character, and the natural order of things. There were moments when some of those I followed seemed to view their lived realities as just the way things were for particular kinds of people in particular kinds of places—a form of "misrecognition" that Bourdieu refers to as symbolic violence. However, concepts like habitus and symbolic violence miss much of the anxious uncertainty and open-endedness that characterized senses of place and self among those I followed. They provide only a partial picture of how young people engaged with the politics of place in Vancouver across time. The historical sediments that constitute the habitus are certainly bound up in the configurations of practices, practical knowledges, and habits of relating that shaped young people's trajectories. However, these trajectories were also inflected by various, and in some cases rapidly changing, technologies (e.g., opioid agonist therapies), political elements (e.g., harm reduction), and local and global imaginaries, resulting in new commonsense understandings of the world that could diverge significantly from past experience.

11. Crack shacks are houses in which drugs are sold and consumed. They are generally run-down and vary significantly depending on how open or closed they are to newcomer customers. While some have the feel of an all-day house party where you can stay as long as you have the money to keep buying, others are accessible only to those with the right connections.

12. Red zones refer to court-mandated spatial restrictions that bar individuals from entering certain neighborhoods.

13. Drug dealing is an extremely broad category. In the context of this project, it could refer to anything from "flipping" small quantities of drugs for minor amounts of profit (which was often immediately used toward supporting one's own substance use) to transporting and selling larger quantities of drugs for one of Greater Vancouver's gangs, which could result in thousands of dollars of profit per week.

PART 2   SOMETHING

1. In describing young people's substance use as a form of vital experimentation, I take inspiration from both Deleuze (2007) and Raikhel and Garriott's (2013b, 26) articulation of addiction as an "experiential and experimental trajectory." As the latter note, addiction can be understood as a way to "harness the experiential or experimental potential of the body by means of a particular substance" (28) as individuals navigate various intimate and institutional domains across time. This experimentation carries tremendous risks, and across this project young people increasingly navigated the interplay between life (the vital) and death (the lethal), even as the forms of experimentation that they were engaged in increasingly included the use of licit pharmacotherapies (Meyers 2013).

2. See also Jason Pine's *The Alchemy of Meth* (2019) and Angela Garcia's *The Pastoral Clinic* (2010) for how substances can generate senses of hope and possibility that punctuate the banal rhythms of the everyday.

3. By 2015 in Greater Vancouver, heroin was heavily adulterated with highly potent, illicitly manufactured fentanyl. I use the term "heroin/fentanyl" to signal this transition.

4. See George Karandinos and others (2014, 9) for a discussion of violent altercations in the context of street-level dealing and crime as "fun, exciting events rife with potential" and Ralph (2014, 17) for a description of injury as "potential, an engine, [and] a generative force that propelled new trajectories."

5. There continues to be significant debate surrounding what constitutes a gang in diverse settings. For those I followed, however, there was no ambiguity surrounding this term. When my interlocutors talked about gangs, they were referring to both the organized crime syndicates that largely control the drug trade in BC (namely, a North American outlaw motorcycle gang and a transnational Chinese gang) and a handful of street gangs, including a well-known Indigenous street gang that originated in eastern Canada. While these local street gangs may have begun as loose groupings of young people formed in high schools and juvenile detention facilities, as they have grown and formed alliances with organized crime syndicates they have also come to play a significant role in large-scale drug trafficking in BC, including across the Canada-U.S. border.

Those I knew were not generally members of these gangs. However, many young men who were involved in dealing and crime were tenuously connected with one of these gangs. These affiliations took the form of street-level subcontract illicit employment (Karandinos et al. 2014); young men described themselves as working for a gang member boss by dealing drugs and committing crimes. They were also frequently subcontracted by gang members—who, it should be noted, were themselves likely very low-level players in gang hierarchies—to engage in robbery and car theft and the delivery of brutal physical punishments related to drug debts and other kinds of heated conflicts. Similar to what has been observed elsewhere (Densley 2013), after an initial period of more close supervision, this kind of loosely gang-connected, street-level dealing and crime was usually carried out quite independently by young men, who could themselves become a boss of sorts to their own set of street-level workers as they were given increasing responsibilities.

While the gangs described above are generally characterized by established leadership and hierarchies among members (Venkatesh 1997), at the street level relationships between gang-member employers and loosely gang-connected, street-level workers were much more ephemeral—collaborations formed and disbanded over time, albeit usually with the same gang.

6. Previous work has described how life on the streets is animated by a moral economy, in which everyday sociability is facilitated through the exchange of goods, services, money, and subcontract illicit employment (Bourgois and Schonberg 2009; Karandinos et al. 2014). Here, I am more concerned with how romantic relationships and low-level, loosely gang-connected dealing and crime opened up a "range of possibilities for morally being in the world and ethically working on oneself" (Zigon 2013, 202), propelling young people forward each day.

7. A fierce commitment to staying together no matter what often clashed with the imperatives of the healthcare, criminal justice, and child protection systems, which frequently man-

dated a separation of young couples for periods of time during pregnancy and early parenting. For example, social workers often dictate that one or both romantic partners attend residential treatment if they want to maintain or regain custody of their child following birth. Due to the lack of residential treatment options that allow young couples to attend together, a decision to attend residential treatment was also often a decision to separate for a period. Like their social workers, the young couples I knew often also envisioned pregnancy and early parenting as times to reduce or eliminate their substance use. Yet when faced with the dilemma of whether or not to separate for a period, many decided that what was right for them was to stay together, even as professionals issued stern warnings that doing so would mean child protective services involvement and most likely permanently losing custody of their child or children. Young people expressed tremendous frustration and a painful sense of confusion regarding the ways that social workers, law enforcement, and other professionals endeavored to break couples apart and did nothing to keep families together because from their perspective this approach was fundamentally wrong.

8. Given the ephemeral quality of relationships between street-level, subcontracted workers and gang member employers, young people's loyalty often seemed to be more to particular moral logics of gang (keeping your mouth shut and going to jail, for example), as opposed to a particular employer with whom they had developed an enduring relationship.

9. Whether they were anchored by romantic relationships, the gang, or something else entirely, the moral worlds that powerfully animated young people's lives cannot be reduced to oppositional value systems forged in the margins. Even the moral logics of the gang, which were sometimes used to make sense of practices that are typically at odds with normative claims of morality—acts of extreme violence, for example—were usually used to convey highly conventional understandings of the good, such as the imperative to protect women and children (see also Henry 2015). Many saw the gang as exacting punishments where the state had failed them. On the streets and in jail, rape and child molestation could get one killed. Extreme acts of violence, when administered according to a strict moral code, lent the gang a sort of ethical superiority to the state for many. This was particularly the case, perhaps, for those many young people whose own abuse had gone unacknowledged by the government or had occurred while they were in government care.

10. Most important to those I knew, it seemed, was that the gang was a site in which the lines around physical violence were clearly drawn and forms of protection were founded and guaranteed. This ethical orientation toward violence as governable seemed to be a comfort to many, for whom chaos and instability had often been the only constants in their lives growing up.

11. Métis scholar Robert Henry (2015) argues that gang activity can allow Indigenous young men to participate in and elaborate particular constructions of masculinity centered on independence and toughness. Participation in gang activity among Indigenous young men both subverts and reinforces settler-colonial logics and projects, however (Henry 2015, 2019). Through the gang, young people reclaim power, strength, urban space, and a clearer path to manhood. Simultaneously, they can reinforce perceptions of Indigenous young people as lawless and violent, increasing their chances of child welfare and criminal justice system involvement.

PART 3   LOST

1. The term "City of Glass" comes from Douglas Coupland (2009).

2. See Marina Morrow and others (2010) for a critical discussion of how the closure of Riverview in the absence of appropriate fiscal arrangements and housing and mental health

supports undermined the promises of a community-based, recovery-oriented model of care and meaningful inclusion for people living with mental illnesses.

3. This report also drew heavily on the findings of the Mental Health Commission of Canada's At Home/Chez Soi study, which was conducted across five major Canadian cities, including Vancouver, between 2010 and 2013 (Currie et al. 2014; Somers et al. 2013). The study consisted of randomly assigning homeless individuals to different treatment options that all included housing (Assertive Community Treatment, intensive case management, and supportive housing) and to a control group described as "treatment as usual," which in Vancouver typically meant homelessness, high rates of police interaction, and sporadic access to basic care. Not surprisingly, the study design was subject to heavy criticism by some local activists, providers, and academics, who were distressed by the fact that people assigned to the control group would continue to live in deplorable conditions while other participants received housing.

4. The BC Mental Health Act is one of the most coercive in all of Canada in terms of how it facilitates the forceful detention and treatment of individuals deemed by police to be "dangerous" and "ill" (Van Veen, Ibrahim, and Morrow 2018). A recent report by the BC Representative for Children and Youth (2021) found that from 2008 to 2018 Mental Health Act apprehensions among children and young people increased from 973 to 2,545, or by 162 percent. While there are insufficient data available, Indigenous young people are almost certainly disproportionately represented in these numbers, given the racism that continues to pervade the criminal justice and healthcare systems in BC (Turpel-Lafond 2020).

5. While young people did not experience the kind of geographical dislocation described by Mindy Fullilove (2005) in her examination of the impacts of urban renewal on African American communities during the second half of the twentieth century, they did experience similar kinds of loss. See also Nicholas Blomley (2014) and Kyle Mays (2016) for discussion of how the disappearance and disconnection of Indigenous people from urban space has long been central to settler-colonial projects in North America.

6. Rundown, privately owned SROs continue to exist in Vancouver's inner city. By referring to a rupture between the old days and the new days, my intention is to reflect young people's colloquial ways of talking about lived experiences of urban change. Viewed from another perspective, the processes of urban change I describe are characterized less by rupture than by incremental shifts toward a new regime of community care—shifts that have by no means encompassed all of Vancouver's SROs or encompassed them to the same degree at the same time (DeVerteuil and Wilton 2009).

7. See Mariana Valverde (2006) for a discussion of how those who are not working in policing or private security may be co-opted into the surveillance and regulation of people who inhabit the margins of society.

8. Contingency management is a behavioral therapy that uses tangible rewards to help a person achieve desired behaviors, including abstinence from substance use. At St. Mary's and Northwest Apartments, the program was used with young people to encourage a range of behaviors, from tidying one's room to adhering to opioid agonist therapy.

9. See Christopher Van Veen and others (2018) for a discussion of how coercive psychiatric practices are powerfully gendered and racialized. Indigenous young men like Joe, Aaron, and Terry continue to be overrepresented among those diagnosed with disorders such as schizophrenia and are more likely to be detained under laws such as BC's Mental Health Act.

10. Indigenous young people are vastly overrepresented in Canada's government care and criminal justice systems with devastating effects, leading Indigenous activists, scholars, and others to argue that these systems provide two of the most heinous examples of the colonial present in Canada (Martin and Walia 2019).

11. These experiences contrast with the findings of a study from Baltimore, which demonstrated that urban revitalization could ward off haunting memories (Linton et al. 2013).

12. In her examination of young women of color and the gentrification of the Lower East Side of New York City, Caitlin Cahill (2007) similarly discusses the disorientation these women experienced between feeling stuck in a gritty neighborhood and longing to be incorporated into the glamorous flows of capital that were transforming that neighborhood.

13. Terminal City is a nickname for Vancouver that references its location as the western terminus of the Canadian Pacific Railway.

14. The title of this section comes from David Cunningham (2017).

15. Terry's reflections are supported by local research, which underscores the success of housing first models in improving adherence to antipsychotic medications (and delivering significant cost savings to government as a result) (Rezansoff et al. 2017).

16. These spaces share a striking resemblance with the "more peaceful edge zones of the city" described by Teresa Gowan (2010, 124) in her ethnography of homelessness in San Francisco, where she observed that some recyclers created alternative spaces for themselves far removed from the "homeless archipelago" of the Tenderloin district.

17. From 2011 to 2015 I collaborated with young people on a photo essay project that examined their senses of place in the city across time. From 2015 to 2018 there were a number of public exhibits featuring the images that individuals had produced (see Fast 2017).

PART 4 NOWHERE

1. Saltwater City is a name for Vancouver used by early Chinese migrants to the city (Yee 2006).

2. See Henry (2019) for a discussion of how tagging and other kinds of physical markings reflect an elaborate street politics of recognition among young Indigenous gang members, asserting their presence and legacy within and across urban neighborhoods. Among those I followed, notions of carrying on or leaving behind a legacy were often charged with momentum—one that could perhaps endure even after death.

3. Withdrawal management has been associated with elevated risks of HIV and hep C transmission and overdose and nearly universal relapse when implemented without plans for transition to longer-term treatments such as OAT (MacArthur et al. 2014; Strang et al. 2003).

4. Research indicates that buprenorphine (one component of Suboxone along with naloxone) has a safety profile six times greater than methadone in terms of overdose risk. Notably, it causes less respiratory depression than methadone and has also been associated with improved educational and employment outcomes, lower relapse rates, higher retention rates, and lower likelihood of misuse (Bell et al. 2009; Fudala et al. 2003; Johnson et al. 2000; Kakko et al. 2003; Maremmani and Gerra 2010; Marsch et al. 2005).

However, research also demonstrates that methadone may support greater treatment retention when compared to buprenorphine (Minozzi et al. 2014) and in particular among individuals who are using opioids intensively (Proctor et al. 2014). Buprenorphine may simply not "hold them" (prevent cravings and withdrawal symptoms), and they generally feel better on high doses of methadone or slow-release oral morphine.

5. iOAT was officially available to those over eighteen and unofficially available to younger individuals based on a physician's discretion. Prescription hydromorphone and dextroamphetamine were made available in the spring of 2020 in an attempt to mitigate the risks of the dual public health emergencies of COVID-19 and overdose. These prescriptions were intended to provide people who use drugs with a safer supply of opioids and stimulants, reducing the

risks of cravings, withdrawal, and overdose at a time when people were being asked to socially distance and self-isolate (BC Centre on Substance Use 2020).

6. Surveys of adolescents with substance use disorders and in treatment for substance use have found that many (approximately 63 to 64 percent) have a concurrent psychiatric disorder of varying severity (Bukstein and Horner 2010; Grella, Joshi, and Rounds-Bryant 2001; Hser et al. 2001). Teasing out the relationship between substance use disorders and some psychiatric disorders can be challenging. Notably, it can be extraordinarily difficult to distinguish between a primary psychiatric disorder such as schizophrenia and recurrent episodes of stimulant-induced psychosis among young people who have used meth intensively for a number of years (Bramness et al. 2012; Fluyau, Mitra, and Lorthe 2019; Glasner-Edwards and Mooney 2014). Many of those I followed had used meth daily for a number of years and seemed to move fairly regularly in and out of periods of psychosis, confounding the DSM-5 definition of substance-induced psychosis as persisting for less than one month after acute substance intoxication or withdrawal.

7. The label "antipsychotics" can be misleading in terms of how these drugs are actually used. For example, some second- and third-generation antipsychotics are prescribed to treat bipolar, mood, anxiety, and sleep disorders among young people (Di Pietro and Illes 2015; Murphy et al. 2015). In the case of those I followed, they were often navigating recurrent episodes of stimulant-induced psychosis and one or more of these disorders.

8. There are ongoing concerns about the appropriateness of OAT for young people who have been using opioids for relatively short periods prior to treatment yet will likely be on (and off) OAT for long periods given the lifelong nature of this treatment for many patients (Fischer 2000; Ranjan, Pattanayak, and Dhawan 2014). It has been argued that there is a large population of young opioid users in Canada for whom alternative treatment modalities (for example, psychosocial treatment combined with medication-assisted detoxing and tapering) may be more appropriate than longer-term pharmacotherapies (Bickel et al. 1997; Sees et al. 2000). Alternatively, others have highlighted the hazards of these treatment modalities in the context of the current overdose crisis and argued strongly for the lifesaving potential of longer-term OAT for young people (Borodovsky et al. 2018; Hadland, Wood, and Levy 2016; Matson et al. 2014).

9. When compared to methadone or slow-release oral morphine, buprenorphine tends to promote greater abstinence from illicit opioids because it has a high affinity for the mμ receptor, which means that it reduces the effects of additional opioid use (Whelan and Remski 2012).

10. Scaling up this kind of interdisciplinary, team-based approach is a key priority in BC (Government of BC 2019). This approach has been demonstrated to be particularly effective in treating and promoting recovery among young people experiencing opioid use disorders (Cottrill and Matson 2014; Guarino et al. 2009; Hopfer, Khuri, and Crowley 2003).

11. The "chronic and relapsing brain disease" model of addiction, which establishes an expectation of relapse, can counter stigmatizing discourses that blame people for their drug use and its effects (Campbell 2007). However, as Garcia (2010) has described, it can also create a sense of "unendingness" and inevitable demise among those seeking treatment and actually undermine treatment success (see also Giang et al. 2020; Gonzales et al. 2012).

12. Second-stage recovery houses generally admit individuals who have already completed at least one month of residential treatment.

13. New regulations were introduced in 2019 in an attempt to crack down on what the head of the Ministry of Mental Health and Addictions called the "Wild West" of recovery houses operated across the province (Bramham 2019).

14. See Garcia (2010, 12) for a discussion of how various "dead ends" experienced by the researcher and her research subjects can "provide us with clues to what is most at stake for the subject."

15. Popular representations of meth use found in the media and anti-meth advertising campaigns often aim to underscore the downward spiral of severe harms that can be set in motion by the decision to try meth, even "just once" (Montana Meth Project 2013). In contrast to this, most of those I knew associated a transition to regular meth use with the mediation of numerous harms, especially at first. Positive understandings and experiences of meth were often constructed in relation to understandings and experiences of crack and heroin/fentanyl use (Fast et al. 2014).

16. Many of those I followed were enmeshed in what Lauren Berlant (2011) calls "cruel optimism." As they engaged and disengaged with various housing and treatment interventions, they were increasingly faced with the troubling sense that these interventions would not necessarily produce different, better futures.

17. In her ethnography of machine gambling addiction, Natasha Schüll (2012, 19) describes the "world-dissolving state of subjective suspension and affective calm" that her research subjects derived from entering "the zone" of machine play. For Schüll, machine gambling addiction represents an intensification of Sigmund Freud's death drive, "a set of tendencies whose aim was to extinguish life's excitations and restore stasis" (223). I am documenting something quite different: addiction as a means of amplifying excitement in circumstances frequently marked by boredom, stagnation, and frequent stops and starts.

18. As others have long argued (Bourgois 2000), OAT involves multifarious forms of discipline, including daily trips to the pharmacy for witnessed dosing and regular appointments with a physician for monitoring. While youth-focused in-patient treatment settings in Greater Vancouver vary widely in terms of institutional feel, they include or can be virtually indistinguishable from hospital wards.

19. See Henry (2019) for a related discussion of how Indigenous gangs challenge settler colonialism by claiming and controlling urban space through territorialization.

20. For some, the line of flight (Deleuze and Guattari 1987) was being everywhere and nowhere; they moved constantly in and out of downtown and across the suburbs of Greater Vancouver. For others, the line of flight was to the interstitial urban spaces that continued to form right up against those of intensive intervention.

21. The sense of momentum opened up by intensive drug use was often inextricable from the rich socialities that, as Philippe Bourgois and Jeff Schonberg (2009) have shown, hold together communities of addicted bodies in the margins. Yet my research equally revealed the forms of isolation that can emerge as young people attempted to evade or refuse housing and treatment programs and other interventions.

22. I am not arguing here for increased attention to pleasure in drug research, although such arguments are important (Moore 2008). Rather, I am pointing to the immediate sense of momentum that can be generated by the rhythms and geographies of addiction and how it may be a powerful antidote to the stagnation and stops and starts generated by the churn of intervention, historical oppression, and marginality (Stewart 2007).

23. Affect's political potential has been a focus of much previous anthropological work (see, for example, Ahmed 2010; Garcia 2017; Million 2013; Ralph 2017).

PART 5   EVERYWHERE

1. Vancouver receives on average 1,199 milometers (47.2 inches) of rainfall a year. Especially during the winter months, the city has a reputation for wet weather.

2. While stabilization care admissions could be involuntary, treatment during admissions was voluntary.

AFTERWORD

1. Here again the thinking of Deleuze and Guattari (1987) can be helpful for understanding the spatial dynamics at play. They distinguish between the smooth and heterogeneous spaces desired by the nomad and the striated and homogenous spaces desired by the state. The nomad seeks smooth spaces of movement and possibility, from which new trajectories can emerge. In contrast, the state seeks striated spaces that regulate and discipline movement and possibility. This book demonstrates some of the failures of state efforts to striate urban space and enduring nomadic ambitions to render it smooth. I thank one of the anonymous reviewers of this book for this insight.

REFERENCES

Ahmed, S. 2010. "Happy Objects." In *The Affect Theory Reader*, edited by G. J. Seigworth and M. Gregg, 1–29. Durham, NC: Duke University Press.

Allison, A. 2014. *Precarious Japan*. Durham, NC: Duke University Press.

Amit, V., and N. Dyck, eds. 2006. *Claiming Individuality: The Cultural Politics of Distinction*. London: Pluto Press.

Anderson, C. 2013. "Urban Aboriginality as a Distinctive Identity, in Twelve Parts." In *Indigenous in the City: Contemporary Identities and Cultural Innovation*, edited by E. Peters and C. Anderson, 46–68. Durham, NC: Duke University Press.

Ball, J., and A. Ross. 1991. *The Effectiveness of Methadone Maintenance Treatment: Patients, Programs, Services and Outcomes*. New York: Springer.

Barnes, T., and T. Hutton. 2009. "Situating the New Economy: Contingencies of Regeneration and Dislocation in Vancouver's Inner City." *Urban Studies* 46 (5–6): 1247–1269.

Barrie, J. M. 2004. *Peter Pan*. 7th ed. New York: Penguin.

BC Centre for Disease Control. 2021. "Toward the Heart: BCCDC Harm Reduction Services." https://towardtheheart.com.

BC Centre on Substance Use. 2018. "Treatment of Opioid Use Disorder for Youth Guideline Supplement." https://www.bccsu.ca/care-guidance-publications.

———. 2020. "Risk Mitigation in the Context of Dual Public Health Emergencies." https://www.bccsu.ca/risk-mitigation-in-the-context-of-dual-public-health-emergencies-v1-5/.

BC Centre on Substance Use and BC Ministry of Health. 2017. "A Guideline for the Clinical Management of Opioid Use Disorder." https://www.bccsu.ca/care-guidance-publications.

BC Coroners Service. 2018. "Child Mortality in British Columbia." https://www2.gov.bc.ca/gov/content/life-events/death/coroners-service/statistical-reports.

———. 2022. "Illicit Drug Toxicity Deaths in BC January 1, 2012–December 31, 2022." https://www2.gov.bc.ca/assets/gov/birth-adoption-death-marriage-and-divorce/deaths/coroners-service/statistical/illicit-drug.pdf

BC Housing. 2019a. "Supportive Housing." https://www.bchousing.org/housing-assistance/housing-with-support/supportive-housing.

BC Housing. 2019b. "SRO Renewal Initiative." https://www.infrastructurebc.com/projects/operational-complete/sro-renewal-initiative.

BC Ministry of Housing and Social Development. 2008. "Unique Partnership Formed at Government SRO Hotels." https://archive.news.gov.bc.ca/releases/news_releases_2005-2009/2008hsd0095-001569.htm.

BC Representative for Children and Youth. 2015. "Paige's Story: Abuse, Indifference and a Young Life Discarded." https://rcybc.ca/wp-content/uploads/2019/05/rcy-pg-report-final.pdf.

———. 2021. "Detained: Rights of Children and Youth under the Mental Health Act." https://rcybc.ca/reports-and-publications/detained/.

Bell, J. R., B. Butler, A. Lawrance, R. Batey, and P. Salmelainen. 2009. "Comparing Overdose Mortality Associated with Methadone and Buprenorphine Treatment." *Drug and Alcohol Dependence* 104 (1): 73–77.

Bellett, G. 2013. "Vancouver Police Mental Health Team Tries to Stop the Revolving Door of Arrest and Treatment. *Vancouver Sun*, April 24, 2013. https://vancouversun.com/health

/mental%20health/vancouver-police-mental-health-team-tries-to-stop-the-revolving
-door-of-arrest-and-treatment.

Bengtsson, T. T. 2012. "Boredom and Action: Experiences from Youth Confinement." *Journal of Contemporary Ethnography* 41 (5): 526–553.

Berlant, L. 2011. *Cruel Optimism*. Durham, NC: Duke University Press.

Bickel, W. K., L. Amass, S. T. Higgins, G. J. Badger, and R. A. Esch. 1997. "Effects of Adding Behavioral Treatment to Opioid Detoxification with Buprenorphine." *Journal of Consulting and Clinical Psychology* 65 (5): 803–810.

Biehl, J. 2005. *Vita: Life in a Zone of Social Abandonment*. Berkeley: University of California Press.

———. 2013. "Ethnography in the Way of Theory." *Cultural Anthropology* 28 (4): 573–597.

Biehl, J., and P. Locke. 2017a. "The Anthropology of Becoming." In *Unfinished: The Anthropology of Becoming*, edited by J. Biehl and P. Locke, 41–89. Durham, NC: Duke University Press.

———. 2017b. *Unfinished: The Anthropology of Becoming*. Durham, NC: Duke University Press.

Blomley, N. 2008. "Enclosure, Common Right and the Property of the Poor." *Social and Legal Studies* 17 (3): 311–331.

———. 2014. *Unsettling the City: Urban Land and the Politics of Property*. New York: Routledge.

Boilevin, L., J. Chapman, L. Deane, C. Doerksen, G. Fresz, D. J. Joe, N. Leech-Crier, S. Marsh, J. McLeod, S. Neufeld, S. Pham, L. Shaver, P. Smith, M. Steward, D. Wilson, and P. Winter. 2018. "Research 101: A Manifesto for Ethical Research in the Downtown Eastside." http://bit.ly/R101Manifesto.

Borodovsky, J. T., S. Levy, M. Fishman, and L. A. Marsch. 2018. "Buprenorphine Treatment for Adolescents and Young Adults with Opioid Use Disorders: A Narrative Review." *Journal of Addiction Medicine* 12 (3): 170–183.

Bourdieu, P. 1977. *Outline of a Theory of Practice*. Cambridge: Cambridge University Press.

———. 1997. *Pascalian Meditations*. Stanford, CA: Stanford University Press.

Bourgois, P. 1996. *In Search of Respect: Selling Crack in El Barrio*. Cambridge: Cambridge University Press.

———. 2000. "Disciplining Addictions: The Bio-politics of Methadone and Heroin in the United States." *Culture, Medicine and Psychiatry* 24 (2): 165–195.

Bourgois, P., and J. Schonberg. 2009. *Righteous Dopefiend*. Berkeley: University of California Press.

Boyd, J., D. Cunningham, S. Anderson, and T. Kerr. 2016. "Supportive Housing and Surveillance." *International Journal of Drug Policy* 34:72–79.

Boyd, J., and T. Kerr. 2016. "Policing 'Vancouver's Mental Health Crisis': A Critical Discourse Analysis." *Critical Public Health* 26 (4): 418–433.

Boyd, S., D. MacPherson, and B. Osborn. 2009. *Raise Shit! Social Action Saving Lives*. Winnipeg: Fernwood.

Bramham, D. 2019. "B.C. Addictions Minister Targets Province's 'Wild, Wild West' Recovery Houses." *Vancouver Sun*, August 23, 2019. https://vancouversun.com/opinion/columnists/daphne-bramham-b-c-addictions-minister-targets-provinces-wild-wild-west-recovery-houses.

Bramness, J. G., O. H. Gunderson, J. Guterstam, E. B. Rognli, E. M. Loberg, S. Medhus, L. Tanum, and J. Franck. 2012. "Amphetamine-Induced Psychosis—A Separate Diagnostic Entity or Primary Psychosis Triggered in the Vulnerable?" *BioMed Central Psychiatry* 12 (1): 221.

Brissett, D., and R. P. Snow. 1993. "Boredom: Where the Future Isn't." *Symbolic Interaction* 16 (3): 237–256.

Brodwin, P. 2011. "Futility in the Practice of Community Psychiatry." *Medical Anthropology Quarterly* 25 (2): 189–208.

Bukstein, O. G., and M. S. Horner. 2010. "Management of the Adolescent with Substance Use Disorders and Comorbid Psychopathology." *Child and Adolescent Psychiatric Clinics* 19 (3): 609–623.

Cahill, C. 2007. "Negotiating Grit and Glamour: Young Women of Color and the Gentrification of the Lower East Side." *City and Society* 19 (2): 202–231.

Campbell, N. 2007. *Discovering Addiction: The Science and Politics of Substance Abuse Research.* Ann Arbor: University of Michigan Press.

Canêdo, J., K. Sedgemore, K. Ebbert, H. Anderson, R. Dykeman, K. Kincaid, C. Dias, D. Silva, Youth Health Advisory Council, R. Charlesworth, R. Knight, and D. Fast. 2022. "Harm Reduction Calls to Action from Young People Who Use Drugs on the Streets of Vancouver and Lisbon." *Harm Reduction Journal* 19 (1): 1–8.

Castañeda, Q. E. 2005. "Between Pure and Applied Research: Experimental Ethnography in a Transcultural Tourist Art World." *National Association for the Practice of Anthropology Bulletin* 23 (1): 87–118.

City of Vancouver. 2014. "Caring for All: Priority Actions to Address Mental Health and Addictions." https://canadacommons.ca/artifacts/1186201/caring-for-all/1739325/.

———. 2023. "Supportive Housing for Homeless and At-Risk Residents." https://vancouver .ca/people-programs/supportive-housing.aspx.

Cohen, A. 2001. "The Search for Meaning: Eventfulness in the Lives of Homeless Mentally Ill Persons in the Skid Row District of Los Angeles." *Culture, Medicine and Psychiatry* 25: 277–296.

Collier, S. J., and A. Lakoff. 2005. "On Regimes of Living." In *Global Assemblages: Technology, Politics and Ethics as Anthropological Problems*, edited by A. Ong and S. J. Collier, 22–39. Oxford: Blackwell.

Comaroff, J., and J. L. Comaroff. 2000. "Millennial Capitalism: First Thoughts on a Second Coming." *Public Culture* 12 (2): 291–343.

Cottrill, C. B., and S. C. Matson. 2014. "Medication-Assisted Treatment of Opioid Use Disorder in Adolescents and Young Adults." *Adolescent Medicine: State of the Art Reviews* 25 (2): 251–265.

Coulthard, G. 2010. "Place against Empire: Understanding Indigenous Anti-colonialism." *Affinities: A Journal of Radical Theory, Culture, and Action*, November 23, 2010. https://ojs .library.queensu.ca/index.php/affinities/article/view/6141.

———. 2014. *Red Skin, White Masks: Rejecting the Colonial Politics of Recognition.* Minneapolis: University of Minnesota Press.

Coupland, D. 2009. *City of Glass: Douglas Coupland's Vancouver.* Vancouver: Douglas & McIntyre.

Culhane, D. 2003. "Their Spirits Live within Us: Aboriginal Women in Downtown Eastside Vancouver Emerging into Visibility." *American Indian Quarterly* 27 (3/4): 593–606.

———. 2003/2004. "Domesticated Time and Restricted Space: University and Community Women in Downtown Eastside Vancouver." *BC Studies* 140: 91–106.

———. 2005. "Representing Downtown Eastside Vancouver." *BC Studies* 147:109–113.

———. 2011. "Stories and Plays: Ethnography, Performance and Ethical Engagements." *Anthropologica* 53 (2): 257–274.

Currie, L. B., A. Moniruzzaman, M. L. Patterson, and J. M. Somers. 2014. "At Home / Chez Soi Project: Vancouver Site Final Report." Mental Health Commission of Canada. https://mentalhealthcommission.ca/resource/vancouver-final-report-at-home-chez-soi -project/.

Das, V., and D. Poole, eds. 2004. *Anthropology in the Margins of the State*. Santa Fe: School of American Research Press.

Davila, A. 2003. "Dreams of Place: Housing, Gentrification, and the Marketing of Space in El Barrio." *Centro Journal* 15 (1): 112.

Deleuze, G. 1995. *Negotiations, 1972–1990*. New York: Columbia University Press.

———. 1997. *Essays Critical and Clinical*. Minneapolis: University of Minnesota Press.

———. 2006. *Two Regimes of Madness: Texts and Interviews 1975–1995*. Los Angeles: Semiotext(e).

———. 2007. "Two Questions on Drugs." In *Two Regimes of Madness*, edited by D. Lapoujade, 151–155. Cambridge, MA: MIT Press.

Deleuze, G., and F. Guattari. 1987. *A Thousand Plateaus: Capitalism and Schizophrenia*. Minneapolis: University of Minnesota Press.

Densley, J. A. 2013. *How Gangs Work: An Ethnography of Youth Violence*. Oxford: Palgrave Macmillan.

DeVerteuil, G. 2003. "Homeless Mobility, Institutional Settings, and the New Poverty Management." *Environment and Planning A: Economy and Space* 35 (2): 361–379.

DeVerteuil, G., and R. Wilton. 2009. "Spaces of Abeyance, Care and Survival: The Addiction Treatment System as a Site of 'Regulatory Richness.'" *Political Geography* 28 (8): 463–472.

Di Pietro, N., and J. Illes. 2015. *The Science and Ethics of Antipsychotic Use in Children*. Amsterdam: Elsevier.

Dorries, H. 2019. "'Welcome to Winnipeg': Making Settler Colonial Urban Space in 'Canada's Most Racist City.'" In *Settler City Limits: Indigenous Resurgence and Colonial Violence in the Urban Prairie West*, edited by H. Dorries et al., 25–43. Winnipeg: University of Manitoba Press.

———. 2023. "Indigenous Urbanism as an Analytic: Towards Indigenous Urban Theory." *International Journal of Urban and Regional Research* 47 (1): 110–118.

Dorries, H., R. Henry, D. Hugill, T. McCreary, and J. Tomiak, eds. 2019. *Settler City Limits: Indigenous Resurgence and Colonial Violence in the Urban Prairie West*. Winnipeg: University of Manitoba Press.

Downtown Eastside Street Market Society. 2014. "Downtown Eastside Street Market Brochure." https://dtesvancouver.com/uploads/curriculum-vitae/109-cv-1627365999.pdf.

Dreifuss, J. A., M. L. Griffin, K. Frost, G. M. Fitzmaurice, J. Sharpe-Potter, D. A. Fiellin, J. Selzer, M. Hatch-Maillette, S. C. Sonne, and R. D. Weiss. 2013. "Patient Characteristics Associated with Buprenorphine/Naloxone Treatment Outcome for Prescription Opioid Dependence: Results from a Multisite Study." *Drug and Alcohol Dependence* 131 (1–2): 112–118.

Drug Users' Liberation Front. n.d. "Dope on Arrival Program." Vancouver. https://www.dulf.ca/doa.

Economist Intelligence Unit. 2022. "The Global Liveability Index 2022." https://www.eiu.com/n/campaigns/global-liveability-index-2022/.

Elliott, D. 2014. "Truth, Shame, Complicity, and Flirtation: An Unconventional, Ethnographic (Non)Fiction." *Anthropology and Humanism* 39 (2): 145–158.

Elliott, D., M. Krawcyzk, C. Gurney, A. Myran, R. Rockthunder, and L. Storm. 2015. "Reimagining Aboriginality, Addictions, and Collaborative Research in Inner City Vancouver, Canada." *Creative Approaches to Research* 8 (1): 22.

Ericson, R. V., and K. D. Haggerty. 1997. *Policing the Risk Society*. Toronto: University of Toronto Press.

Fanon, F. 2008. *Black Skin, White Masks*. New York: Grove Press.

Farmer, P. 2004. *Pathologies of Power: Health, Human Rights, and the New War on the Poor.* Vol. 4. Berkeley: University of California Press.

Fast, D. 2016. "'My Friends Look Just Like You': Research Encounters and Imaginaries in Vancouver's Urban Drug Scene." *Medicine Anthropology Theory* 3 (2) :223–243.

———. 2017. "Dream Homes and Dead Ends in the City: A Photo Essay Experiment." *Sociology of Health and Illness* 39 (7): 1134–1148.

———. 2021. "Going Nowhere: Ambivalence about Drug Treatment during an Overdose Public Health Emergency in Vancouver." *Medical Anthropology Quarterly* 35 (2): 209–225.

Fast, D., T. Kerr, E. Wood, and W. Small. 2014. "The Multiple Truths about Crystal Meth among Young People Entrenched in an Urban Drug Scene: A Longitudinal Ethnographic Investigation." *Social Science and Medicine* 110 (0): 41–48.

Fast, D., J. Shoveller, and T. Kerr. 2017. "The Material, Moral, and Affective Worlds of Drug Dealing and Crime among Young Men Entrenched in an Inner City Drug Scene." *International Journal of Drug Policy* 44:1–11.

Fast, D., J. Shoveller, K. Shannon, and T. Kerr. 2009. "Safety and Danger in Downtown Vancouver: Understandings of Place among Young People Entrenched in an Urban Drug Scene." *Health and Place* 16 (1): 51–60.

Fast, D., J. Shoveller, W. Small, and T. Kerr. 2013. "Did Somebody Say Community? Young People's Critiques of Conventional Community Narratives in the Context of a Local Drug Scene." *Human Organization* 72 (2): 98–110.

First Nations Health Authority. 2015. "#itstartswithme. FNHA's Policy Statement on Cultural Safety and Humility." https://www.fnha.ca/documents/fnha-policy-statement-cultural-safety-and-humility.pdf.

———. 2017. "Overdose Data and First Nations in BC: Preliminary Findings." https://www2.gov.bc.ca/assets/gov/overdose-awareness/fnha_overdosedataandfirstnationsinbc_preliminary findings_finalweb_july20.pdf.

Fischer, B. 2000. "Prescriptions, Power and Politics: The Turbulent History of Methadone Maintenance in Canada." *Journal of Public Health Policy* 21 (2): 187–210.

Fischer, B., P. Kurdyak, E. Goldner, M. Tyndall, and J. Rehm. 2016. "Treatment of Prescription Opioid Disorders in Canada: Looking at the 'Other Epidemic'?" *Substance Abuse Treatment, Prevention, and Policy* 11 (1): 1.

Fischer, M. 2003. *Emergent Forms of Life and the Anthropological Voice.* Durham, NC: Duke University Press.

Fluyau, D., P. Mitra, and K. Lorthe. 2019. "Antipsychotics for Amphetamine Psychosis: A Systematic Review." *Frontiers in Psychiatry* 10:740.

Foucault, M. 1997a. "Technologies of the Self." In *Ethics: Subjectivity and Truth,* edited by P. Rabinow, 223–251. New York: Free Press.

———. 1997b. "The Birth of Biopolitics." In *Ethics: Subjectivity and Truth,* edited by P. Rabinow, 73–79. New York: Free Press.

Fudala, P. J., T. P. Bridge, S. Herbert, W. O. Williford, C. N. Chiang, K. Jones, J. Collins, D. Raisch, P. Casadonte, J. Goldsmith, W. Ling, U. Malkerneker, L. McNicholas, J. Renner, S. Stine, and D. Tusel for the Buprenorphine/Naloxone Collaborative Study Group. 2003. "Office-Based Treatment of Opiate Addiction with a Sublingual-Tablet Formulation of Buprenorphine and Naloxone." *New England Journal of Medicine* 349 (10): 949–958.

Fullilove, M. 2005. *Root Shock: How Tearing Up City Neighborhoods Hurts America, and What We Can Do about It.* New York: One World.

Garcia, A. 2008. "The Elegiac Addict: History, Chronicity, and the Melancholic Subject." *Cultural Anthropology* 23 (4): 718–746.

―――. 2010. *The Pastoral Clinic: Addiction and Dispossession along the Rio Grande*. Berkeley: University of California Press.

―――. 2017. "Heaven." In *Unfinished: The Anthropology of Becoming*, edited by J. Biehl and P. Locke, 111–129. Durham, NC: Duke University Press.

German, D., and C. Latkin. 2012. "Boredom, Depressive Symptoms, and HIV Risk Behaviors among Urban Injection Drug Users." *AIDS and Behavior* 16 (8): 2244–2250.

Giang, V., M. Thulien, R. McNeil, K. Sedgemore, H. Anderson, and D. Fast. 2020. "Opioid Agonist Therapy Trajectories among Street Entrenched Youth in the Context of a Public Health Crisis." *Social Science and Medicine–Population Health* 11:100609.

Glasner-Edwards, S., and L. J. Mooney. 2014. "Methamphetamine Psychosis: Epidemiology and Management." *Central Nervous System Drugs* 28 (12): 1115–1126.

Gomart, E. 2002. "Towards Generous Constraint: Freedom and Coercion in a French Addiction Treatment." *Sociology of Health and Illness* 24 (5): 517–549.

Gonzales, R., D. Anglin, R. Beattie, C. A. Ong, and D. C. Glik. 2012. "Perceptions of Chronicity and Recovery among Youth in Treatment for Substance Use Problems." *Journal of Adolescent Health* 51 (2): 144–149.

Goodfellow, A. 2008. "Pharmaceutical Intimacy: Sex, Death, and Methamphetamine." *Home Cultures* 5 (3): 271–300.

Goodman, A., K. Fleming, N. Marwick, T. Morrison, L. Lagimodiere, T. Kerr, and Western Aboriginal Harm Reduction Society. 2017. "'They Treated Me Like Crap and I Know It Was Because I Was Native': The Healthcare Experiences of Aboriginal Peoples Living in Vancouver's Inner City." *Social Science and Medicine* 178:87–94.

Goodstein, E. S. 2005. *Experience Without Qualities: Boredom and Modernity*. Stanford, CA: Stanford University Press.

Goodyear, T., S. Robinson, E. Jenkins, M. Gagnon, K. Mitchell, and R. Knight. 2021. "Involuntary Stabilization Care of Youth Who Overdose: A Call for Evidence- and Ethics-Informed Substance Use Policy." *Canadian Journal of Public Health* 112 (3): 456–459.

Gordillo, G. 2004. *Landscape of Devils: Tensions of Place and Memory in the Argentinean Chaco*. Durham, NC: Duke University Press.

Gordon, A. F. 2008. *Ghostly Matters: Haunting and the Sociological Imagination*. Minneapolis: University of Minnesota Press.

Government of BC. 2019. "A Pathway to Hope: A Roadmap for Making Mental Health and Addictions Care Better for People in British Columbia." https://www2.gov.bc.ca/assets /gov/british-columbians-our-governments/initiatives-plans-strategies/mental-health -and-addictions-strategy/bcmentalhealthroadmap_2019web-5.pdf.

―――. 2020a. "Community Care and Assisted Living Act." https://www.bclaws.gov.bc.ca /civix/document/id/complete/statreg/00_02075_01.

―――. 2020b. "Mental Health Act." https://www.bclaws.gov.bc.ca/civix/document/id /complete/statreg/96288_01.

―――. 2021a. "Agreements with Youth Adults." https://www2.gov.bc.ca/gov/content/family -social-supports/youth-and-family-services/teens-in-foster-care/agreements-with -young-adults.

―――. 2021b. "Youth Agreements." https://www2.gov.bc.ca/gov/content/safety/public -safety/protecting-children/youth-agreements.

Gowan, T. 2010. *Hobos, Hustlers and Backsliders*. Minneapolis: University of Minnesota Press.

Grella, C. E., V. Joshi, and J. Rounds-Bryant. 2001. "Drug Treatment Outcomes for Adolescents with Comorbid Mental and Substance Use Disorders." *Journal of Nervous and Mental Disease* 189 (6): 384–392.

Guarino, H. M., L. A. Marsch, L. W. S. Campbell, S. P. Gargano, D. L. Haler, and R. Solhkhah. 2009. "Methadone Maintenance Treatment for Youth: Experiences of Clients, Staff, and Parents." *Substance Use and Misuse* 44 (14): 1979–1989.

Hadland, S. E., E. Wood, and S. Levy. 2016. "How the Pediatric Workforce Can Address the Opioid Crisis." *Lancet* 388 (10051): 1260.

Hammond, C. J. 2016. "The Role of Pharmacotherapy in the Treatment of Adolescent Substance Use Disorders." *Child and Adolescent Psychiatric Clinics* 25 (4): 685–711.

Hansen, H. 2018. *Addicted to Christ: Remaking Men in Puerto Rican Pentecostal Drug Ministries.* Berkeley: University of California Press.

Harris, C. 2002. *Making Native Space: Colonialism, Resistance and Reserves in British Columbia.* Vancouver: University of British Columbia Press.

Henry, R. 2015. "Social Spaces of Maleness: The Role of Street Gangs in Practising Indigenous Masculinities." In *Indigenous Men and Masculinities: Legacies, Identities, Regeneration,* edited by R. A. Innes and K. Anderson, 181–196. Winnipeg: University of Manitoba Press.

———. 2019. "'I Claim in the Name of . . .': Indigenous Street Gangs and the Politics of Recognition in Prairie Cities." In *Settler City Limits: Indigenous Resurgence and Colonial Violence in the Urban Prairie West,* edited by H. Dorries et al., 222–247. Winnipeg: University of Manitoba Press.

Hopfer, C. J., E. Khuri, and T. J. Crowley. 2003. "Treating Adolescent Heroin Use." *Journal of the American Academy of Child and Adolescent Psychiatry* 42 (5): 609–609.

Hser, Y. I., C. E. Grella, R. L. Hubbard, S. C. Hsieh, B. W. Fletcher, B. S. Brown, and M. D. Anglin. 2001. "An Evaluation of Drug Treatments for Adolescents in 4 US Cities." *Archives of General Psychiatry* 58 (7): 689–695.

Jervis, L. L., P. Spicer, and S. M. Manson. 2003. "Boredom, 'Trouble,' and the Realities of Postcolonial Reservation Life." *Ethos* 31 (1): 38–58.

Johnson, R. E., M. A. Chutuape, E. C. Strain, S. L. Walsh, M. L. Stitzer, and G. E. Bigelow. 2000. "A Comparison of Levomethadyl Acetate, Buprenorphine, and Methadone for Opioid Dependence." *New England Journal of Medicine* 343 (18): 1290–1297.

Kakko, J., K. D. Svanborg, M. J. Kreek, and M. Heilig. 2003. "1-Year Retention and Social Function after Buprenorphine-Assisted Relapse Prevention Treatment for Heroin Dependence in Sweden: A Randomised, Placebo-Controlled Trial." *Lancet* 361 (9358): 662–668.

Karandinos, G., L. K. Hart, F. M. Castrillo, and P. Bourgois. 2014. "The Moral Economy of Violence in the US Inner City." *Current Anthropology* 55 (1): 1–22.

Killaspy, H., S. Kingett, P. Bebbington, R. Blizard, S. Johnson, F. Nolan, S. Pilling, and M. King. 2009. "Randomised Evaluation of Assertive Community Treatment: 3-Year Outcomes." *British Journal of Psychiatry* 195 (1): 81–82.

Knight, K. R. 2015. *Addicted. Pregnant. Poor.* Durham, NC: Duke University Press.

Lavalley, J., S. Kastor, J. Valleriani, and R. McNeil. 2018. "Reconciliation and Canada's Overdose Crisis: Responding to the Needs of Indigenous Peoples." *Canadian Medical Association Journal* 190 (50): E1466–E1467.

Ley, D. 2012. "Social Mixing and the Historical Geography of Gentrification." In *Mixed Communities: Gentrification by Stealth?,* edited by G. Bridge, T. Butler, and L. Lees, 53–68. Bristol: Policy Press.

Linton, S. L., C. E. Kennedy, C. A. Latkin, D. D. Celentano, G. D. Kirk, and S. H. Mehta. 2013. "'Everything That Looks Good Ain't Good!' Perspectives on Urban Redevelopment among Persons with a History of Injection Drug Use in Baltimore, Maryland." *International Journal of Drug Policy* 24 (6): 605–613.

Liu, S., and N. Blomley. 2013. "Making News and Making Space: Framing Vancouver's Downtown Eastside." *Canadian Geographer* 57 (2): 119–132.

López, A. M. 2020. "Necropolitics in the 'Compassionate' City: Care/Brutality in San Francisco." *Medical Anthropology* 39 (8): 1–14.

López, A. M., M. Abbey-Bey, and T. Spellman. 2018. "Resisting Overdose." *Anthropology News* 59 (1): 50–56.

Lorway, R. 2021. "Remembering HIV in the Era of Eradication: Critical Nostalgia, Infrastructures of Accountability, and the Fate of Viral Socialities." In *Living with HIV in "Post-crisis" Times: Beyond the Endgame,* edited by D. A. B. Murray, 215-226. London: Lexington Books.

Lupick, T. 2017. *Fighting for Space.* Vancouver: Arsenal Pulp Press.

MacArthur, G. J., E. van Velzen, N. Palmateer, J. Kimber, A. Pharris, V. Hope, A. Taylor, K. Roy, E. Aspinall, D. Goldberg, T. Rhodes, D. Hedrich, M. Salminen, M. Hickman, and S. J. Hutchinson. 2014. "Interventions to Prevent HIV and Hepatitis C in People Who Inject Drugs: A Review of Reviews to Assess Evidence of Effectiveness." *International Journal of Drug Policy* 25 (1): 34–52.

Mahmood, S. 2005. *Politics of Piety: The Islamic Revival and the Feminist Subject.* Princeton, NJ: Princeton University Press.

Mains, D. 2012. *Hope Is Cut: Youth, Unemployment, and the Future in Urban Ethiopia.* Philadelphia: Temple University Press.

Maremmani, I., and G. Gerra. 2010. "Buprenorphine-Based Regimens and Methadone for the Medical Management of Opioid Dependence: Selecting the Appropriate Drug for Treatment." *American Journal on Addictions* 19 (6): 557–568.

Marsch, L. A., W. K. Bickel, G. J. Badger, M. E. Stothart, K. J. Quesnel, C. Stanger, and J. Brooklyn. 2005. "Comparison of Pharmacological Treatments for Opioid-Dependent Adolescents: A Randomized Controlled Trial." *Archives of General Psychiatry* 62 (10): 1157–1164.

Martin, C. M., and H. Walia. 2019. "Red Women Rising: Indigenous Women Survivors in Vancouver's Downtown Eastside." Downtown Eastside Women's Centre. https://dewc.ca/resources/redwomenrising.

Masquelier, A. 2019. *Fada: Boredom and Belonging in Niger.* Chicago: University of Chicago Press.

Massey, D. 1994. *Space, Place, and Gender.* Minneapolis: University of Minnesota Press.

Massumi, B. 2002. *Parables for the Virtual: Movement, Affect, Sensation.* Durham, NC: Duke University Press.

Matson, S. C., G. Hobson, M. Abdel-Rasoul, and A. E. Bonny. 2014. "A Retrospective Study of Retention of Opioid-Dependent Adolescents and Young Adults in an Outpatient Buprenorphine/Naloxone Clinic." *Journal of Addiction Medicine* 8 (3): 176–182.

Mays, K. T. 2016. "Pontiac's Ghost in the Motor City: Indigeneity and the Discursive Construction of Modern Detroit." *Middle West Review* 2 (2): 115–142.

McCann, E. J. 2008. "Expertise, Truth, and Urban Policy Mobilities: Global Circuits of Knowledge in the Development of Vancouver, Canada's 'Four Pillar' Drug Strategy." *Environment and Planning A: Economy and Space* 40 (4): 885–904.

McConville, B. J., and M. T. Sorter. 2004. "Treatment Challenges and Safety Considerations for Antipsychotic Use in Children and Adolescents with Psychoses." *Journal of Clinical Psychiatry* 65 (4): 20–29.

Mehta, A., and L. Bondi. 1999. "Embodied Discourse: On Gender and Fear of Violence." *Gender, Place and Culture* 6 (1): 67–84.

Meyers, T. 2013. *The Clinic and Elsewhere: Addiction, Adolescents, and the Afterlife of Therapy.* Seattle: University of Washington Press.

Million, D. 2013. *Therapeutic Nations: Healing in an Age of Indigenous Human Rights.* Tucson: University of Arizona Press.

Minozzi, S., L. Amato, C. Bellisario, and M. Davoli. 2014. "Maintenance Treatments for Opiate-Dependent Adolescents." *Cochrane Database of Systematic Reviews* 6.

Mirabal, N. R. 2009. "Geographies of Displacement: Latina/os, Oral History, and the Politics of Gentrification in San Francisco's Mission District." *Public Historian* 31 (2): 7–31.

Moakley, P. 2021. "The 'Safe Supply' Movement Aims to Curb Drug Deaths Linked to the Opioid Crisis." *Time*, October 25, 2021. https://time.com/6108812/drug-deaths-safe-supply -opioids/.

Montana Meth Project. 2013. "Montana Meth Project." https://montanameth.org.

Montaner, J. S. G., R. Hogg, E. Wood, T. Kerr, M. Tyndall, A. R. Levy, and P. R. Harrigan. 2006. "The Case for Expanding Access to Highly Active Antiretroviral Therapy to Curb the Growth of the HIV Epidemic." *Lancet* 368 (9534): 531–536.

Monture, P. A. 2007. "Race and Erasing: Law and Gender in White Settler Societies." In *Race and Racism in 21st Century Canada*, edited by S. P. Heir and B. S. Bolaria, 197–216. Peterborough: Broadview Press.

Moore, D. 2008. "Erasing Pleasure from Public Discourse on Illicit Drugs: On the Creation and Reproduction of an Absence." *International Journal of Drug Policy* 19 (5): 353–358.

Morrow, M., P. K. B. Dagg, and A. Pederson. 2008. "Is Deinstitutionalization a 'Failed Experiment'? The Ethics of Re-institutionalization." *Journal of Ethics in Mental Health* 3 (2): 1–7.

Morrow, M., J. Smith, A. Pederson, L. Battersby, V. Josewski, and B. Jamer. 2010. *Relocating Mental Health Care in British Columbia: Riverview Hospital Redevelopment, Regionalization and Gender in Psychiatric and Social Care*. Vancouver: Centre for the Study of Gender, Social Inequities and Mental Health.

Mullins, G. (Host). 2022. "Episode 31: Love, Death, and Benzodope." *Crackdown Podcast*, April 22, 2022. https://www.crackdownpod.com/episodes/31-lovedeathbenzodope.

Murphy, A. L., D. M. Gardner, S. Kisely, C. Cooke, S. P. Kutcher, and J. Hughes. 2015. "A Qualitative Study of Antipsychotic Medication Experiences of Youth." *Journal of the Canadian Academy of Child and Adolescent Psychiatry* 24 (1): 61–69.

Murray, K. B. 2011. "Making Space in Vancouver's East End: From Leonard Marsh to the Vancouver Agreement." *BC Studies* 169:7–49.

———. 2015. "Bio-gentrification: Vulnerability Bio-Value Chains in Gentrifying Neighbourhoods." *Urban Geography* 36 (2): 277–299.

Musharbash, Y. 2007. "Boredom, Time, and Modernity: An Example from Aboriginal Australia." *American Anthropologist* 109 (2): 307–317.

Netherland, J., and H. B. Hansen. 2016. "The War on Drugs That Wasn't: Wasted Whiteness, 'dirty Doctors,' and Race in Media Coverage of Prescription Opioid Misuse." *Culture, Medicine, and Psychiatry* 40 (4): 664–686.

Neufeld, S. D., J. Chapman, N. Crier, S. Marsh, J. McLeod, and L. A. Deane. 2019. "Research 101: A Process for Developing Local Guidelines for Ethical Research in Heavily Researched Communities." *Harm Reduction Journal* 16 (1): 1–11.

Nguyen, V. K. 2010. *The Republic of Therapy*. Durham, NC: Duke University Press.

Nosyk, B., R. S. Joe, J. S. G. Montaner, and E. Wood. 2014. "On the Successes of the BC Opioid Substitution Treatment System, and How We Can Build upon Them." *British Columbia Medical Journal* 56 (10): 510–513.

O'Neill, B. 2014. "Cast Aside: Boredom, Downward Mobility, and Homelessness in Postcommunist Bucharest." *Cultural Anthropology* 29 (1): 8–31.

Oppal, W. T. 2012. "Forsaken: The Report of the Missing Women Commission of Inquiry." Vancouver: Missing Women Commission of Inquiry. https://www2.gov.bc.ca/assets/gov /law-crime-and-justice/about-bc-justice-system/inquiries/forsaken-es.pdf.

Paul, B., M. Thulien, R. Knight, M. J. Milloy, B. Howard, S. Nelson, and D. Fast. 2020. "'Something That Actually Works': Cannabis Use among Young People in the Context of Street Entrenchment." *PLOS ONE* 15 (7): e0236243.

Pearce, M. E., K. A. Jongbloed, C. G. Richardson, E. W. Henderson, S. D. Pooyak, E. Oviedo-Joekes, W. M. Christian, M. T. Schechter, and P. Spittal, for the Cedar Project Partnership. 2015. "The Cedar Project: Resilience in the Face of HIV Vulnerability within a Cohort Study Involving Young Indigenous People Who Use Drugs in Three Canadian Cities." *BioMed Central Public Health* 15 (1): 1095.

Pels, P. 1999. "Professions of Duplexity." *Current Anthropology* 40 (2): 101–114.

Peters, E., and C. Anderson, eds. 2013. *Indigenous in the City: Contemporary Identities and Cultural Innovation*. Vancouver: University of British Columbia Press.

Petryna, A. 2002. *Life Exposed: Biological Citizens after Chernobyl*. Princeton, NJ: Princeton University Press.

Phillips, S. D., B. J. Burns, E. R. Edgar, K. T. Mueser, K. W. Linkins, R. A. Rosenheck, R. E. Drake, and E. C. McDonel-Herr. 2001. "Moving Assertive Community Treatment into Standard Practice." *Psychiatric Services* 52 (6): 771–779.

Pilarinos, A., P. Kendall, D. Fast, and K. DeBeck. 2018. "Secure Care: More Harm Than Good." *Canadian Medical Association Journal* 190 (41): E1219–E1220.

Pine, J. 2019. *The Alchemy of Meth: A Decomposition*. Minneapolis: University of Minnesota Press.

Preble, E., and J. J. Casey. 1969. "Taking Care of Business: The Heroin User's Life on the Street." *Substance Use & Misuse* 4 (1): 1–24.

Proctor, S. L., A. Copeland, A. M. Kopak, P. L. Herschman, and N. Polukhina. 2014. "A Naturalistic Comparison of the Effectiveness of Methadone and Two Sublingual Formulations of Buprenorphine on Maintenance Treatment Outcomes: Findings from a Retrospective Multisite Study." *Experimental and Clinical Psychopharmacology* 22 (5): 424.

Providence Health Care. 2016. "Addiction Medicine Consult Team (AMCT) at St. Paul's Hospital." https://familymedicine.providencehealthcare.org/programs/addiction-medicine.

———. 2020. "Rapid Access Addiction Clinic (RAAC)." https://www.providencehealthcare.org/rapid-access-addiction-clinic-raac.

Raikhel, E., and W. Garriott, eds. 2013a. *Addiction Trajectories*. Durham, NC: Duke University Press.

———. 2013b. "Introduction: Tracing New Paths in the Anthropology of Addiction." In *Addiction Trajectories*, edited by E. Raikhel and W. Garriot, 8–56. Durham, NC: Duke University Press.

Ralph, L. 2014. *Renegade Dreams: Living through Injury in Gangland Chicago*. Chicago: University of Chicago Press.

———. 2017. "Becoming Aggrieved: An Alternative Framework of Care in Black Chicago." In *Unfinished: The Anthropology of Becoming*, edited by J. Biehl and P. Locke, 93–110. Durham, NC: Duke University Press.

Ralph, M. 2008. "Killing Time." *Social Text* 26 (4): 1–29.

Ranjan, R., R. D. Pattanayak, and A. Dhawan. 2014. "Long-Term Agonist and Antagonist Therapy for Adolescent Opioid Dependence: A Description of Two Cases." *Indian Journal of Psychological Medicine* 36 (4): 439–443.

Razack, S. 2007. "When Place Becomes Race." In *Race and Racialization: Essential Readings*, edited by T. D. Gupta et al., 74–82. Toronto: Canadian Scholars' Press.

———. 2015. *Dying from Improvement: Inquest and Inquiries into Indigenous Deaths*. Toronto: University of Toronto Press.

Rezansoff, S. N., A. Moniruzzaman, S. Fazel, L. McCandless, R. Procyshyn, and J. M. Somers. 2017. "Housing First Improves Adherence to Antipsychotic Medication among Formerly Homeless Adults with Schizophrenia: Results of a Randomized Controlled Trial." *Schizophrenia Bulletin* 43 (4): 852–861.

Robbins, J. 2013. "Beyond the Suffering Subject: Toward an Anthropology of the Good." *Journal of the Royal Anthropological Institute* 19 (3): 447–462.

Robertson, L. A. 2006. "Risk, Citizenship, and Public Discourse: Coeval Dialogues on War and Health in Vancouver's Downtown Eastside." *Medical Anthropology* 25 (4): 297–330.

———. 2007. "Taming Space: Drug Use, HIV, and Homemaking in Downtown Eastside Vancouver." *Gender, Place and Culture* 14 (5): 527–549.

Roe, G. 2009/2010. "Fixed in Place: Vancouver's Downtown Eastside and the Community of Clients." *BC Studies* 164:75–101.

Roitman, J. 2005. "The Garrison-Entrepot: A Mode of Governing in the Chad Basin." In *Global Assemblages: Technology, Politics and Ethics as Anthropological Problems*, edited by A. Ong and S. J. Collier, 417–436. Malden, MA: Blackwell.

Scheper-Hughes, N., and P. Bourgois. 2003. "Introduction: Making Sense of Violence." In *Violence in War and Peace: An Anthology*, edited by N. Scheper-Hughes and P. Bourgois, 1–31. Hoboken, NJ: John Wiley.

Schüll, N. D. 2012. *Addiction by Design: Machine Gambling in Las Vegas*. Princeton, NJ: Princeton University Press.

Schuman-Olivier, Z., R. D. Weiss, B. B. Hoeppner, J. Borodovsky, and M. J. Albanese. 2014. "Emerging Adult Age Status Predicts Poor Buprenorphine Treatment Retention." *Journal of Substance Abuse Treatment* 47 (3): 202–212.

Sees, K. L., K. L. Delucchi, C. Masson, A. Rosen, H. W. Clark, H. Robillard, P. Banys, and S. M. Hall. 2000. "Methadone Maintenance vs 180-Day Psychosocially Enriched Detoxification for Treatment of Opioid Dependence: A Randomized Controlled Trial." *Journal of the American Medical Association* 283 (10): 1303–1310.

Shuman, A. 2006. "Entitlement and Empathy in Personal Narrative." *Narrative Inquiry* 16 (1): 148–155.

Simpson, A. 2014. *Mohawk Interruptus: Political Life across the Borders of Settler States*. Durham, NC: Duke University Press.

Somers, J. M., M. L. Patterson, A. Moniruzzaman, L. Currie, S. N. Rezansoff, A. Palepu, and K. Fryer. 2013. "Vancouver At Home: Pragmatic Randomized Trials Investigating Housing First for Homeless and Mentally Ill Adults." *Trials* 14 (1): 365.

Sterk, C. E. 1999. *Fast Lives: Women Who Use Crack Cocaine*. Philadelphia: Temple University Press.

Stevenson, L. 2014. *Life Beside Itself*. Oakland: University of California Press.

Stewart, K. 2007. *Ordinary Affects*. Durham, NC: Duke University Press.

Stewart, M., and C. La Berge. 2019. "Care-to-Prison Pipeline: Indigenous Children in Twenty-First-Century Settler Colonial Economies." In *Settler City Limits: Indigenous Resurgence and Colonial Violence in the Urban Prairie West*, edited by H. Dorries et al., 196–221. Winnipeg: University of Manitoba Press.

Strang, J., J. McCambridge, D. Best, T. Beswick, J. Bearn, S. Rees, and M. Gossop. 2003. "Loss of Tolerance and Overdose Mortality after Inpatient Opiate Detoxification: Follow Up Study." *BioMed Central* 326 (7396): 959–960.

Stueck, W. 2006. "Group Protests Vanishing Housing." *Globe and Mail*, October 23, 2006. https://www.theglobeandmail.com/news/national/group-protests-vanishing-housing/article654503/.

Sue, K. 2019. *Getting Wrecked: Women, Incarceration, and the American Opioid Crisis*. Berkeley: University of California Press.

Thompson, S. 2010. "Policing Vancouver's Mentally Ill: The Disturbing Truth: Update." Vancouver Police Department. https://vpd.ca/wp-content/uploads/2021/06/vpd-lost-in-transition-part-2.pdf.

Thulien, M., H. Anderson, S. Douglas, R. Dykeman, A. Horne, B. Howard, K. Sedgemore, R. Charlesworth, and D. Fast. 2022. "The Generative Potential of Mess in Community-Based Participatory Research with Young People Who Use(d) Drugs in Vancouver." *Harm Reduction Journal* 19 (1): 1–13.

Todd, Z. 2019. "Decolonizing Prairie Public Art: The Further Adventures of the Ness Namew." In *Settler City Limits: Indigenous Resurgence and Colonial Violence in the Urban Prairie West*, edited by H. Dorries et al., 25–43. Winnipeg: University of Manitoba Press.

Tomiak, J. 2019. "Contested Entitlement: The Kapyong Barracks, Treaty Rights, and Settler Colonialism in Winnipeg." In *Settler City Limits: Indigenous Resurgence and Colonial Violence in the Urban Prairie West*, edited by H. Dorries et al., 95–117. Winnipeg: University of Manitoba Press.

Tsing, A. 2005. *Friction: An Ethnography of Global Connection*. Princeton, NJ: Princeton University Press.

Tuck, E. 2009. "Suspending Damage: A Letter to Communities." *Harvard Educational Review* 79 (3): 409–428.

Turpel-Lafond, M. E. 2020. "In Plain Sight: Addressing Indigenous-Specific Racism and Discrimination in B.C. Health Care." https://engage.gov.bc.ca/addressingracism/.

Udechuku, A., J. Olver, K. Hallam, F. Blyth, M. Leslie, M. Nasso, P. Schlesinger, L. Warren, M. Turner, and G. Burrows. 2005. "Assertive Community Treatment of the Mentally Ill: Service Model and Effectiveness." *Australasian Psychiatry* 13 (2): 129–134.

Valverde, M. 2006. *Law and Order: Images, Meanings, Myths*. New Brunswick, NJ: Rutgers University Press.

Vancouver Agreement. 2010. "Vancouver Agreement: 2000–2010 Highlights." Province of BC, Government of Canada.

Vancouver Coastal Health Authority. 2023a. "Downtown Eastside Second Generation Health System Strategy." https://www.vch.ca/en/downtown-eastside-2nd-generation-strategy#:~:text=The%20new%20model%20brings%20together,all%20available%20at%20one%20site.

———. 2023b. "Community-Based Mental Health & Substance Use Services." https://www.vch.ca/en/health-topics/community-based-mental-health-substance-use-services.

———. 2023c. "Vancouver Community's Child &Youth Mental Health & Substance Use Strategy." https://www.vch.ca/en/vancouver-communitys-child-youth-mental-health-substance-use-strategy.

———. 2023d. "Addiction Medicine at Downtown Eastside Connections Clinic." https://www.vch.ca/en/location-service/addiction-medicine-downtown-eastside-connections-clinic.

Vancouver Police Department. 2009. "Project Lockstep: A United Effort to Save Lives in the Downtown Eastside." https://vpd.ca/wp-content/uploads/2021/06/vpd-project-lockstep.pdf.

———. 2013. "Vancouver's Mental Health Crisis: An Update Report." https://vpd.ca/wp-content/uploads/2021/06/mental-health-crisis.pdf.

Van Veen, C., M. Ibrahim, and M. Morrow. 2018. "Dangerous Discourses: Masculinity, Coercion, and Psychiatry." In *Containing Madness: Gender and "Psy" in Institutional Contexts*, edited by J. M. Kilty and E. Dej, 241–265. London: Palgrave Macmillan.

Van Veen, C., K. Teghtsoonian, and M. Morrow. 2019. "Enacting Violence and Care: Neoliberalism, Knowledge Claims, and Resistance." In *Madness, Violence, and Power: A Critical Collection*, edited by A. Daley, L. Costa, and P. Beresford, 63–79. Toronto: University of Toronto Press.

Venkat, B. J. 2016. "Cures." *Public Culture* 28:475–497.

Venkatesh, S. A. 1997. "The Social Organization of Street Gang Activity in an Urban Ghetto." *American Journal of Sociology* 103 (1): 82–111.

Vitellone, N. 2004. "Habitus and Social Suffering: Culture, Addiction and the Syringe." *Sociological Review* 52:129–147.

Vo, H. T., E. Robbins, M. Westwood, D. Lezama, and M. Fisherman. 2016. "Relapse Prevention Medications in Community Treatment for Young Adults with Opioid Addiction." *Substance Abuse* 37 (3): 392–397.

Wacquant, L. 2008. *Urban Outcasts: A Comparative Sociology of Advanced Marginality.* Cambridge: Polity.

Warshawski, T., and C. Warf. 2019. "It Is Time for an Ethical, Evidence-Based Approach to Youth Presenting to the ED with an Opioid Overdose." *Paediatrics & Child Health* 24 (6): 374–376.

Whelan, P., and K. Remski. 2012. "Buprenorphine vs Methadone Treatment: A Review of Evidence in Both Developed and Developing Worlds." *Journal of Neurosciences in Rural Practice* 3 (1): 45–50.

Williams, R. 2015. "Structures of Feeling." In *Structures of Feeling: Affectivity and the Study of Culture,* edited by D. Sharma and F. Tygstrup, 20–28. Berlin: De Gruyter.

Wilson-Bates, F. 2008. "Lost in Transition: How a Lack of Capacity in the Mental Health System Is Failing Vancouver's Mentally Ill and Draining Police Resources." Vancouver Police Department. https://vpd.ca/wp-content/uploads/2021/06/vpd-lost-in-transition-part-2.pdf.

Winters, K., E. Tanner-Smith, E. Bresani, and K. Meyers. 2014. "Current Advances in the Treatment of Adolescent Drug Use." *Adolescent Health, Medicine and Therapeutics* 5 (12): 199–210.

Woolford, A. 2001. "Tainted Space: Representations of Injection Drug-Use and HIV/AIDS in Vancouver's Downtown Eastside." *BC Studies* 129 (1): 27–50.

Yee, P. 2006. *Saltwater City: Story of Vancouver's Chinese Community.* Vancouver: Douglas & McIntyre.

Zigon, J. 2013. "On Love: Remaking Moral Subjectivity in Postrehabilitation Russia." *American Ethnologist* 40 (1): 201–215.

INDEX

Page numbers in *italics* refer to illustrative matter.

ABOUT THE AUTHOR

DANYA FAST is an assistant professor in the Department of Medicine (Division of Social Medicine) at the University of British Columbia (UBC) and an associate member of UBC's Department of Anthropology. She is also a research scientist at the British Columbia Centre on Substance Use.

Available titles in the Medical Anthropology:
Health, Inequality, and Social Justice series

Printed and bound by CPI Group (UK) Ltd, Croydon, CR0 4YY

27/10/2024

14580230-0002